Dr. Yadro Ducic MD completed medical school and Head and Neck Surgery training in Ottawa and Toronto, Canada and finished Facial Plastic and Reconstructive Surgery at the University of Minnesota. He moved to Texas in 1997 running the Department of Otolaryngology and Facial Plastic Surgery at JPS Health Network in Fort Worth, and training residents through the University of Texas Southwestern Medical Center in Dallas, Texas. He was a full Clinical Professor in the Department of Otolaryngology-Head Neck Surgery. Currently, he runs a tertiary referral practice in Dallas-Fort Worth. He is Director of the Baylor Neuroscience Skullbase Program in Fort Worth, Texas and the Director of the Center for Aesthetic Surgery. He is also the Codirector of the Methodist Face Transplant Program and the Director of the Facial Plastic and Reconstructive Surgery Fellowship in Dallas-Fort Worth sponsored by the American Academy of Facial Plastic and Reconstructive Surgery. He has authored over 160 publications, being on the forefront of clinical research in advanced head and neck cancer and skull base surgery and reconstruction. He is devoted to advancing the care of this patient population.
For more information please go to www.drducic.com.

Dr. Moustafa Mourad completed his surgical training in Head and Neck Surgery in New York City from the New York Eye and Ear Infirmary of Mt. Sinai. Upon completion of his training he sought out specialization in facial plastic, skull base, and reconstructive surgery at Baylor All Saints, under the mentorship and guidance of Dr. Yadranko Ducic. Currently he is based in New York City as the Division Chief of Head and Neck and Skull Base Surgery at Harlem Hospital, in addition to being the Director for the Center of Aesthetic Surgery in New York. Dr. Mourad is a prolific writer with more than 40 publications in the peer reviewed literature centered around clinical, epidemiological, and translational research. Dr. Mourad is also the founder for the Society for Head and Neck Reconstructive and Microsurgery, dedicated to the advancement and training of future reconstructive surgeons.

Katrina Jensen has been practicing exclusively in the field of Head & Neck rehabilitation for 20 years, including a 4 year training fellowship with the surgeons from the University of Pittsburgh. Throughout her career, she has focused on improving rehabilitative care standards for head & neck cancer patients, working with the American Speech, Language & Hearing Association to improve training standards and clinical practice guidelines within this population. She is currently the Director of Medical Speech Pathology services for Texas Health Care where she has developed and now maintains a very active Head & Neck rehabilitation program, including the largest laryngectomy support group in North Texas. In 2010, she founded a non-profit organization, The North Texas Laryngectomy Society, which serves to benefit laryngeal cancer survivorship. In 2011, she launched PracticalSLPinfo.com, a comprehensive interactive website resource for topics within medical speech pathology. In 2013, she published *The Modern Laryngectomy* which serves as the only comprehensive text on laryngectomy care and rehabilitation. Katrina also conducts practices and research surrounding gastroesophageal/laryngopharyngeal reflux and radiation care for swallow preservation as it pertains to our patient population. She currently is grant funded through a Cancer Prevention & Research collaboration with MD Anderson, to investigate radiation care within the head & neck population. Throughout her career, Katrina has lectured extensively in the fields of laryngectomy rehabilitation as well as medically based voice & swallowing disorders. She's known both nationally and internationally for her expertise in these fields and frequently provides consultative services to similar programs, both in the US as well as abroad.

Table of Contents

What is Head and Neck Cancer? 7

Members of the Management Team 8
   Head and Neck Surgeon 8
   Reconstructive and Plastic Surgeons 9
   Oral and Maxillofacial Surgeon 10
   Radiation and Medical Oncologists 11
   Speech and Swallow Therapists 12

Oral Cancer 13

Oropharyngeal Cancer 21

Nasopharyngeal Cancer 29

Hypopharyngeal Cancer 36

Laryngeal Cancer 43

Nasal and Sinus Cancer 52

Skin Cancer 61

Salivary Gland Malignancies 67

Thyroid Cancer 75

Tracheal Tumors 82

Radiation Treatment 87

Chemotherapy and Other Anti-Tumor Medications 90

Swallowing During Radiation Treatment 96
Keep Swallowing! 96
Exercise Your Swallow 96
Jaw Stretches 96
What to Eat 97
Ouch! When it Hurts to Swallow 97
"I Don't Have an Appetite" 98
Nothing Tastes Right 98
Xerostomia 98
Swallowing with Xerostomia 99
Compensating for Xerostomia 99

Eating by Mouth 101
What to Eat 101
How Much Should I Eat? 102
How Often? 102

Water/Hydration 102

Frequently Asked Questions 103

I know it's important to keep swallowing during radiation but is there a certain amount I should be sure to eat each day?..103
When will I feel the effects of radiation? 103
How long will it take to recover from radiation?..103
Why is my mouth so dry?...103
When will my sense of taste return? 103
Why do I have so much mucous?...104

Why Feeding Tubes are Used 105
Post-operative Recovery 105
Ongoing Cancer Treatment 105
Dysphagia...105

Types of Feeding Tubes 106
Nasogastric Tubes (NG Tube) 106
Gastrostomy Tubes (G-Tube) 106
Jejunostomy Tubes (J-Tube) 106

Enteral Feeding Methods.. 107
Feeding Tube Food..107
Feeding Tube Pumps...107
Gravity Bags 107
Bolus Feeding 107

Gastrostomy Tube Troubleshooting.. 108
Pain At The Tube Site...108
Broken End Tips..108
Clogged or Slow Passage..108

Frequently Asked Questions 108
What is a Feeding Tube?..108
Can I still eat by mouth if I have a feeding tube?..109
If I can eat by mouth, why do I need a feeding tube? 109
Why am I being changed from an NG tube to a G-tube? 109
Can I shower/bathe with a G-tube or J-tube?..109
When can my g-tube be removed? 109

Normal Swallowing 110

Dysphagia 111

Common Symptoms of Dysphagia 112

Evaluating Dysphagia 112
Fiberoptic Endoscopic Examination of Swallowing (FEES)..112
Modified Barium Swallow..113
Clinical Swallow Examination 113

Management of Dysphagia... 113
Dietary Guidelines..114
Intake Modifications...114

Dysphagia Therapy 114
Strength and Range of Motion Exercises...115

Neuromuscular Electrical Stimulation 115

Therapeutic Progress 116

Returning to Eating Again 116

Dietary Guidelines 117

SOFT DIET 117
What is a soft diet? 117
Helpful Hints 117
Foods to AVOID 117

PUREED DIET 118
What is a pureed diet? 118
How do I make pureed foods? 118
Foods to Avoid 118

MOIST DIET 118
What is a moist diet? 118
Helpful Hints 119
Foods to AVOID 119

Thickening Liquids at Home 120
Thickening Agents 120
Levels of Thickened Liquid 120
What Should Be Thickened 120
Things to Avoid 121

THERAPEUTIC FEEDING 121
What/How to Eat 121

Trismus Management 123
Prevention 123
Therapy 124
    Therabite.. *124*
    Dynasplint *124*
Botox 124
Surgery 125

Affected structures 126

Treatment/Therapy 127

Phonation: Not Just the Vocal Cords 128

How a Voice is Produced 128

Dysphonia: When Hoarseness Should Be Addressed 129

Evaluating Voice Changes 130
Stroboscopy...130
Vocal Parameters 131

Types of Voice Disorders 131

Organic Disorders 131

Structural: 131
Neurogenic: 131

Functional Disorders 132

Management of Voice Issues 132
Voice Therapy 132
Medical Management 133
Surgery 133

Common Voice Disorders Following Cancer Treatment: 134

Vocal Fold Paralysis vs. Fixation 134
Paralysis/Paresis 134
Fixation 135

Treatment for Vocal Fold Paralysis/Paresis/Fixation 135
Voice Therapy 135
Vocal Fold Augmentation 135
Medialization Thyroplasty 136

Potential Radiation Changes to Vocal Cords/Larynx 136
Laryngeal Webbing 136
Treatment for Webbing 137
Radiation Fibrosis 137
Treatment for Radiation Fibrosis 137
Radiation Scarring 137
Treatment for Radiation Scarring 137

Vocal Hygeine: Caring for your Voice 138

Vocal Hygiene Protocol 138

Indications 140

Tracheotomy vs Tracheostomy 140
Tracheotomy Procedure 140

Trach Tube Anatomy 101 141
Face Plate 141
Outer Cannula 141
Inner Cannula 141
Shaft 141
Curvature 141
Cuff 142
Pilot Balloon 142
Fenestration(s) 142

Tracheostomy Tube Varieties 143
Cuffed vs Cuffless Tubes 143
Types of Cuffs 143
High Volume/Low Pressure 143
Low Volume/High Pressure 144
Proper Cuff Inflation 144
Assessing Cuff Status 145

Fenestrated vs. Non-Fenestrated Tubes 145

Being a "Neck Breather" 147

Physiologic/Functional Changes 147
Smelling..147
Tasting..147
Coughing...148
Filtration...148
Humidification 148
Speaking..149
Swallowing 149

Speaking with a Tracheostomy Tube 149
Understanding How a Voice is Produced 149
DEFLATE THE CUFF!!! 150
Finger Occlusion 150
Speaking Valves 150
    Passy-Muir Speaking Valve (PMV) 150
Shikani Speaking Valve 152
Specialty Tubes 152

Swallowing with a Tracheostomy 152
Subglottic Pressurization 152
Hyolaryngeal Movement 153

Suction 153

Tracheostomy Care 154
Tracheostomy Site..154
Potential Signs of Infection..154
Cleaning 155

Decannulation 155
Weaning 155
Capping Trials 156
Tube Removal and Wound Care...156

Accidental Decannulation 157

Anatomical Changes 158

Being a "Neck Breather" 158

Functional Changes 159
Communication After Surgery 159

Other Effects of Your Surgery 161

Stoma Care.. 161

Using Suction 162

Bathing and Water Activities 162

Swallowing After Laryngectomy 163

Smelling after Laryngectomy 164

Tracheoesophageal Voice Prosthesis (TEP) 164

Cleaning Your Voice Prosthesis 165

Using an Adhesive Housing 165

Using an HME Cassette 165
Proper Use of an HME Cassette 166
Cleaning Mucous From An HME 167

Larytube Use and Cleaning 167

TEPs and HME's During Radiation Treatment 168
Voice Prostheses During Radiation..168
HME Use During Radiation 168

Laryngectomy FAQs... 168
Why am I coughing so much mucous?...168
When can I get a TEP?...169
How often/when do I use and HME?..169
How often do I replace my HME cassette?...169
When do I use my Larytube? 169
I can't wear my adhesive housing during radiation so how do I continue wearing my HME cassette?..170
Is it ok to wear my adhesive/HME during hyperbaric oxygen treatments?...................170
Can I keep my voice prosthesis if I am going to have hyperbaric oxygen treatments?..........170
Why do I need to change my HME cassette every 24 hours? 170
How often do I change my adhesive housing? 170
Why can't I smell?..170
Why can't I taste my food like I used to? 171
Why is it harder to swallow? 171

What is Head and Neck Cancer?

Cancer is defined as the abnormal growth of cells (tumor) within the body. The behavior of these tumors are variable and are based on the cell origin (pathology), the location of origin, and other patient risk factors. These tumors can be benign with relatively indolent courses, or they may be malignant with a highly aggressive course. It is important to understand the pathology of the diagnosis as this has huge implications in the treatment and prognosis of these lesions.

Cancer of the head and neck is unique from other cancers. The head and neck region is a complex landscape responsible for assisting in many basic human functions. Treatment of head and neck lesions, whether surgically or medically, may compromise an individual's ability to speak, swallow, or breath, as well as potentially impacting their physical appearance. Due to the complexity of the anatomical region, and the variability in the different sites in which cancer occurs, it is important to understand the exact type of cancer, and the site of localization. Before embarking on a treatment plan, the patient should be well versed in the impact it will have on function and quality of life. Often times, treatment requires the involvement of physical therapists, speech pathologists, dentists, and voice specialists to maximize patient outcomes and enhance quality of life.

Members of the Management Team

Overview

The diagnosis, treatment, and management of head and neck cancer requires the coordinated efforts of many specialized healthcare providers. This multidisciplinary team consists of head and neck surgeons, reconstructive and plastic surgeons, oromaxillofacial surgeons, radiation and medical oncologists, and speech and swallow therapists. These members come together to form the core team insuring the best possible outcomes, as well as managing quality of life issues after treatment of a devastating illness.

Head and Neck Surgeon

Head and Neck Surgeons are individuals who have completed residency training in Otolaryngology-Head and Neck Surgery (OHNS) accredited by the Accreditation Counseling for Graduate Medical Education (ACGME). This 5-year training begins after medical school, and is highly structured providing the foundation for their surgical career. In order to be accredited as a Head and Neck Surgeon, physicians need only to complete their training in OHNS. However, some physicians elect to go on to complete an extra 1-2 years of additional training known as a fellowship. Such fellowships provide more opportunity to refine ones skill in the application of head and neck surgical technique. They may go on to learn other skills including microvascular and reconstructive surgery, transoral robotic surgery, and open skull base. Fellowship is not a mandatory requirement and is highly dependent on the individual training received throughout residency. Fellowship training may be provided through the Advanced Training Council by the American Head and Neck Society (AHNS), or through other programs independent of the society. Each fellowship program provides different experiences and advanced skill sets specific to each institution.

Head and Neck Surgeons are responsible for coordinating the care of the majority of head and neck cancer patients. They often times are the first physician a patient is referred to upon suspicion for a cancer. They will often times complete all initial workup of the patient, including initial physical examination, imaging, and diagnostic procedures. Once a diagnosis of cancer is confirmed, they will coordinate the care and treatment of the patient with other members of the multi-disciplinary team. The surgeon's role includes the surgical management of the patient should treatment require surgery. After surgery, the surgeon is involved in routine patient examination for surveillance purposes. They also help in facilitate other quality of life interventions working closely with speech and swallow therapists, oromaxillofacial surgeons, as well as prosthodontists.

Reconstructive and Plastic Surgeons

Head and neck cancer often requires removal of tumor from the most complex and intricate part of the body responsible for swallowing, breathing, and speaking in addition to having far reaching impact on an individual's physical appearance. The wide variety in the physiological and anatomical landscape of the head and neck makes reconstruction complex and challenging. Often times reconstructive and plastic surgeons with specialized training are required to manage these complex defects.

In order to be qualified as a reconstructive surgeon, one must first have completed an ACGME accredited residency training in either Otolaryngology-Head and Neck Surgery or Integrated Plastics Surgery. Alternatively, some individuals may have completed a General Surgery Residency training program, followed by an ACGME accredited Plastic Surgery Fellowship. Once completed, individuals must seek further training in head and neck reconstructive surgery through a recognized training society. Reconstructive surgery training may be completed through the American Academy of Facial Plastics and Reconstructive Surgery (AAFPRS), the American Head and Neck Society (AHNS), or through the American Society for Reconstructive Microsurgery (ASRM). Each training program provides a unique training experience. Specifically, the AHNS and AAFPRS provide reconstructive training of the Head and Neck only, whereas the ASRM will provide training for reconstruction of the rest of the body (e.g. hand). It is important to recognize these differences, and identify the specific training that your reconstructive surgeon has received.

The reconstructive surgeon is tasked with the management of post surgical defects. Reconstructive options vary depending on location of the defects, size of defects, as well as patient related factors. The surgeon may explore different reconstructive options, and should individualize their treatment for each patient. Surgeon goals are to optimally restore the basic physiological and anatomic processes impacted by the ablation, while maximizing quality of life. Ideal goals are to maintain or restore breathing, speaking, and swallowing functions. However, each disease process is different, and reconstructive goals are tailored to each patient.

Oral and maxillofacial surgeons are surgeons that specialize in the diagnosis, treatment, and management of diseases of the oral cavity, jaw, and face. Because a large proportion of head and neck cancer is localized to the oral cavity and face, these surgeons form an integral part of the team. Their role is imperative in order to maximize functional and aesthetic outcomes in the post surgical patient.

Oral and Maxillofacial surgeons (OMFS) are recognized specialty within Dentistry. In order to complete training in OMFS, surgeons must first complete their training either in Doctor of Dental Surgery (DDS) or Doctor of Medicine in Dentistry (DMD) from a school accredited by the Commission on Dental Accreditation (CODA). Once completed, they must apply for further training in oral and maxillofacial training. Depending on the specific training program, practitioners may complete an additional Medical Degree (MD) as part of their training, or proceed directly to their surgical training. They may also proceed to continued advanced training in craniofacial and microvascular surgery.

The OMFS surgeon is part of the multidisciplinary team, whose role extends to restoration and rehabilitation of patients with diseases that affect the mouth, jaw, face and skull. They provide and manage prosthetics, dental implants, as well as assist in reconstruction.

Both radiation and medical oncologists form an integral part of the multidisciplinary team providing non-surgical options for patients suffering from head and neck cancer. Radiation oncologists are physicians specialized in the use of ionizing radiation delivered to areas affected by disease. Medical oncologists are physician specialists that utilize medications in the treatment of these diseases.

In order to be credentialed as a radiation oncologist, after completing medical school, physicians must complete a 4-year ACGME accredited residency in Radiation Oncology. They must subsequently receive certification by the American Board of Radiology (ABR), American Board of Physician Specialties (ABPS), or American Board of Osteopathic Radiology (ABOR). Radiation oncologists may further seek subspecialty training in radiation oncology of the head and neck. Medical oncologists must first complete an ACGME residency in Internal Medicine and become certified by the American Board of Internal Medicine (ABIM). They must then go on to complete their training in an ACGME fellowship in medical oncology, and pass the Medical Oncology Certification Examination. Once completed, they are qualified to diagnose, treat, and manage many of the oncological processes that affect the head and neck.

Radiation and medical oncologists provide valuable treatments either definitively, adjunctively, or in a palliative setting when dealing with head and neck cancers. Radiation oncologists focus on the use of ionizing radiation delivered directly to tissue in order to remove and treat tumors. Medical oncologists utilize systemic medicines to target distant and regional disease. In patients that are poor surgical candidates, or have advanced local disease, radiation and medical treatments may form the cornerstone of their treatment plans. Other disease pathologies, such as lymphomas, are usually managed through medical treatments as opposed to surgery. These physicians are integral in discussions regarding optimal treatment plans, and exploration of non-surgical options.

Patients suffering from post treatment effects often have compromised speech and swallowing abilities. Speech and swallow therapists assist in rehabilitating patients in order to maximize post treatment quality of life. Speech-Language Pathologists have received master's level training at a university accredited by American Speech-Language-Hearing Association (ASHA). Once credentialed they may elect complete a doctorate Speech Language Pathology.

Speech and Swallow therapists are an integral part of the team. They are involved in the pre-treatment and post-treatment assessment of the patient. They provide valuable insight into the extent of disease and treatment impact on patient's quality of life, performing physical and diagnostic examinations. Surgery and radiation may leave patients severely compromised, and they assist in restoration of functions. They provide physical therapy, and routine examination insuring progression and rehabilitation of the patient.

Oral Cancer

Overview

Oral cancer is a term used to address malignancies in the oral cavity, and is the most common of all head and neck cancers. The oral cavity is the region between an individual's lips and their soft palate. When discussing oral cavity cancer, there are different subsites that may be used to better define the site of location better guiding management decisions: lips, tongue, the alveolus (gums), the buccal mucosa (inner cheek), tongue, floor of mouth, and hard palate. The vast majority of cancer arising in the oral cavity involve the epithelial lining. It is within this lining that the cells begin to abnormally proliferate and replicate causing an overgrowth of cells and subsequent tumors. Not all lesions are malignant, with each type of lesions guided by different managing principles.

Causes. The causes of tumor growth in the oral cavity is likely multifactorial with many contributing factors. Overall, the chronic and long-term use of irritants such as tobacco and alcohol are the leading causes of oral cavity cancers. Other predisposing factors include the use of Betel Nut (prominent in India and Southeastern Asian countries), UV light exposure (lip cancer), marijuana, poor dentition, genetic predisposition, and Human papilloma virus (HPV)

Signs and Symptoms. Oral cavity cancers may present in different forms, but generally speaking they are often times found in earlier stages due to earlier detection by patients or other healthcare providers during routine examinations.

- **Pain.** Frequently patients may present with sores in or around their mouth that are painful and longstanding that do not resolve over time. As lesions increase in size, they may become increasingly painful, and may not respond to normal pain medications.
- **Lesions.** Patients or other healthcare providers (e.g. dentists) may notice a lesion that does not resolve or appear abnormal. These lesions may appear as patches, sores, ulcerations, plaques, or masses. Sores that do not resolve in 2-3 weeks usually require further evaluation by a specialist with potential for further workup.
- **Bleeding.** Bleeding from a site within the oral cavity may be a presenting sign. Often times, chronically irritated skin may bleeding due to infections, chronic irritation (brushing), or dentures. However, bleeding from a particular site or lesion should be evaluated by a specialist.
- **Speaking and Swallowing Difficulties.** The presence of a tumor or lesion often times will impact a patients ability to speak or swallow. As lesions grow in size, patients may find it difficult to open their mouths (trismus), chew, or

move their tongue. Tongue lesions may also impact a patients ability to properly articulate words.

- **Poorly Fitting Dentures.** Patients may find increasing difficulty in the use of dentures. This usually occurs in patients with hard palate lesions that prevent the proper fitting of their dentures.
- **Tooth Problems.** Lesions involving the gum line may result in invasion of the tooth socket. This may cause tooth pain there is involvement of the nerves, or may even cause the tooth to become loose or fall out. Also, a non-healing site of a previously extracted tooth may also be a sign of an underlying cancer.
- **Lump in the Neck.** Rarely cancers of the oral cavity can present as a single or multiple lumps in the neck. These enlarged nodes may be reactive due to tumor or an associated infection, or may be a sign of regionally metastatic disease

Diagnosis and Workup. In addition to routine history and physical examination, the physician may perform ancillary tests and procedures in order to confirm the presence and type of oral cavity cancer, as well as to determine the presence of second primary cancers (SPC) or the spread of malignant disease elsewhere.

- **Biopsy.** Often times the first step in the diagnosis of an oral cavity cancer is to perform a biopsy. Several types of biopsies may be performed, in the clinic or operative setting depending on how easily visualized the lesion is, its size, and patient preferences. Taking a biopsy will confirm the presence of abnormal cells under microscopic view, and is imperative in making the diagnosis of oral cavity cancer.
  - **Incisional Biopsy.** Your physician may perform this by removing a piece of the abnormal appearing tissue allowing for microscopic assessment. Typically, results from a biopsy may take up to 1 week to get final results. Multiple biopsies may be needed if insufficient tissue was previously sampled, or if there are multiple suspicious appearing lesions. This may be performed under local anesthesia in the office, depending on size and location, as well as patient comfort and preference.
  - **Excisional Biopsy:** This is a biopsy in which the whole suspicious lesion is excised with a perimeter of normal tissue and examined. This type of biopsy is not routinely performed, at the risk of removing normal tissue unnecessarily.
  - **Lymph Node Biopsy.** If a patient presents with a neck mass, particularly in the setting of no identifiable oral cavity lesion, the physician may sample tissue from lymph node. There are several types of lymph node biopsy.
    - *Fine Needle Biopsy (FNB).* If the mass can be felt by the clinician, then a small needle can be introduced with an attempt at extracting cells for microscopic assessment. The

appearance of abnormal cells will help support the diagnosis of cancer. Sometimes, not enough cells are extracted, and repeat biopsies may need to be performed. This may also be performed with the help of ultrasound or computed tomography (CT) guidance

- *Core Biopsy (CB).* Similar to the Fine Needle Biopsy, a core biopsy is performed by introducing a larger caliber needle, with extraction of tissue as opposed to cells. This core biopsy allows for extraction of more tissue and can be more useful, but often times not necessary, as an FNB is sufficient. This can also be done with or without ultrasound or CT-guided assistance

- *Operative Biopsy.* If the location of the node is too deep, or not readily felt by a clinician, the surgeon may elect to perform biopsy under general anesthesia in an operating room.

- **Blood Work.** The physician may elect to perform routine blood analysis to assist in determining the presence of oral cavity cancer or other present diseases. Blood work may not be necessary, and the decision to obtain blood work is individualized to every patient.
  - **Liver Function Tests (LFTs):** Can be utilized to determine the presence of concurrent liver disease that may be associated with risk factors for the development of oral cavity cancer (alcohol consumption, hepatitis). Furthermore, abnormal values may indicate the presence of metastatic liver disease.
  - **Complete Blood Count (CBC):** This will identify the presence of any anemia that can sometimes be associated with poor nutrition, or chronic illness.
  - **Nutritional Blood Work:** If a patient seems nutritionally depleted, particularly in advanced cases, the clinician may elect to obtain laboratory work up to measure nutrition markers in the blood work. This may assist in determining if a patient requires supplemental nutrition.

- **Imaging.** Often times a physician may elect to obtain imaging that will help in better understanding the presence of cancer and any other underlying issues. Imaging may be performed of the primary site, or of the general region to better define disease extent. The physician may elect to obtain further imaging in situations in which they are concerned for local invasion (e.g. into bone, muscle, adjacent sites), or regional invasion (to the neck). Imaging is not necessary in the diagnosis of all oral cavity cancers, and the decision to obtain imaging or the type of imaging will be best dictated by each patient's individualized care.
  - **Chest X-rays:** Chest radiography may be obtained in order to define the presence of disease in the lungs. Often times patients with oral cavity cancers, have a longstanding history of smoking, and may have associated lesions in their lungs that should be identified.

- **Computed Tomography (CT)**: CT-Scans usually provide a more detailed image of the head and neck region, identifying parts of the tumor that is not readily seen on exam, as well as the presence of regional disease not readily detected (e.g. in the neck). CT-Scans can be obtained with or without contrast. Given the complexity of the region, usually CT scans are obtained with scans, to help in identify the vascular architecture within the neck. However, this is not always necessary, and CT scans may be obtained without contrast in circumstances that preclude patient receiving contrast (iodine allergies, kidney disease).
- **Magnetic Resonanice Imaging (MRI):** MRI is usually obtained in addition to other imaging studies, and is rarely performed in isolation. MRI is obtained if there is suspicion for advanced involvement of soft tissue (e.g. the eye, or brain), or to determine the status of nerves.
- **18-Fluorodeoxyglucose Positron Emission Tomography (18-FDG PET):** FDG-PET scans may be performed with CT or MRI imaging modalities and are utilized for the identification of regional or distant metastases.
- **Dental X-rays (Panorex)**: Panorex scans may be obtained to determine the status of teeth, gum, or jaw involvement.
- **Ultrasound (US)**: Ultrasound may utilized to better characterize neck masses, or used in conjunction with biopsy techniques. US can indicate suspicious characters of lesions that would direct a physician to more aggressive workup (biopsy, excision).

Type of Cancer. The overwhelming majority of cancers of the oral cavity are squamous cell carcinoma. However there are other cancers that also occur in this region that are on the differential diagnosis that must be considered.

- **Squamous Cell Carcinoma.** The vast majority of oral cavity cancers or squamous cell carcinoma. These cancers involve the malignant transformation of the mucosal lining within the oral cavity.
- **Carcinoma In-Situ.** This refers to the earliest stage of squamous cell carcinoma. This may also be referred to as *severe dysplasia.* It indicates that the abnormal proliferation of cells has not extended beyond the deepest layer of tissue. A diagnosis of carcinoma in-situ may not rule out the presence of full squamous cell carcinoma in other regions. However, this is indicates the earliest stage of cancer, and can be removed prior to further invasion.
- **Salivary Gland Tumors.** The oral cavity houses small salivary glands that can be subject to malignant transformation. These cancers have a distinct behavior different from that of cancer involving the epithelial lining. Distinction is often made on biopsy, with appropriate treatment guidance.
- **Lymphoma.** Lymphoma may present as a lesion in the head and neck, although rare.

- **Mucosal Melanoma.** Melanoma, similar to the type of melanoma found in the skin, may also manifest in the oral cavity. Although rare, this is an important consideration, with impact on treatment decisions and outcomes.
- **Jaw Cancers.** There is a wide range of jaw cancers and cysts that may also present as masses in the oral cavity. Identification of these cancers occurs on physical exam in conjunction with radiological imaging.

Staging of Oral Cavity Cancer. Once the appropriate diagnosis and work up of oral cavity cancer is complete, cancer stage is determined. Currently, the method of staging used is the *American Joint Commission on Cancer (AJCC) Staging Manual* 7th edition.[1] The staging system is broadly referred to the TNM staging system, and is a descriptor of the factors that impact the staging of a cancer

- **Tumor Size (T):** This descriptor is used to categorize the size of the primary tumor.
  - **Tx**: Unable to assess primary tumor. This may be assigned in circumstances in which the primary tumor has not presented itself, but the patient has known lymph node disease
  - **Tis**: This refers to *carcinoma in-situ*, a type of cancer without invasion into the deeper structrues of the lining of the epithelial cells.
  - **T1:** The primary tumor is no greater than 2 cm.
  - **T2:** The primary tumor is between 2-4 cm in greatest dimension
  - **T3:** The pimary tumor is greater than 4 cm in greatest dimension.
  - **T4a:** Moderately advanced local disease. This is used to describe tumors with invasion into local tissues outside the confines of the oral cavity including: facial or cervical skin, the jaw, chin, muscle.
  - **T4b:** Very advanced local disease. This describes tumor that invades vital structures or spaces making eradiction of local disease difficult including: spaces around the muscles that assist in chewing, bones in the skull base, or involvement of the carotid artery (major blood supply to the brain).
- **Nodal Status (N):** This descriptor is used to describe the presence and number of lymph nodes in the neck.
  - **Nx:** Unable to assess nodal disease status.
  - **N0:** Absence of any nodal disease.
  - **N1:** There is one single node on the side of the tumor, no greater than 3 cm in its greatest dimension.
  - **N2a:** There is a single node 3-6 cm on the same side of the tumor.
  - **N2b:** There are multiple nodes on the same side of tumor, non greater than 6 cm in its greatest dimension.
  - **N2c:** Presence of any nodal disease opposite to the side of cancer, or both sides of the neck, but none greater than 6 cm in its greatest dimension.
  - **N3:** Presence of any nodes greater than 6 cm in greatest dimension.
- **Metastatic Disease Status (M):** This is used to describe the presence or absence of distant metastatic disease.

- o **M0:** No evidence of distant metastatic disease.
- o **M1:** Presence of distant metastatic disease.
- **Final Staging.** Once a value is assigned to each descriptor of the TNM cancer system, a final stage will be assigned.

Stage 0	Tis	N0	M0
Stage I	T1	N0	M0
Stage II	T2	N0	M0
	T3	N0	M0
Stage III	T1	N1	M0
	T2	N1	M0
	T3	N1	M0
	T4a	N0	M0
	T4a	N1	M0
Stage IVA	T1	N2	M0
	T2	N2	M0
	T3	N2	M0
	T4a	N2	M0
Stage IVB	Any T	N3	M0
	T4b	Any N	M0
Stage IVC	Any T	Any N	M1

- **Other Considerations.**
  - o **Clinical Staging (cTNM):** The clinical stage refers to staging of the patient prior to treatment based on clinical information (physical exam, radiographic images etc).
  - o **Pathological Staging (pTNM):** If surgical removal of tumor is performed, the pathologist will provide their own staging based on their microscopic and gross examination of all specimens.

Treatment Plan. Depending on the site of disease, the clinical staging, and patient factors (co-morbid health conditions, patient preferences) a patient specific treatment plan should be outlined. Broadly speaking there are 3 types of treatment that can be used in combination or separately depending on the type and stage of cancer. The decision to embark on a particular treatment plan should be made involving a multidisciplinary team of doctors (surgeons, radiation oncologists, and medical oncologists) and the patient. Patient specific goals and outcomes should be defined, with a thorough discussion of the risks, benefits, and alternatives of all the separate treatment types.

- **Surgery.** Surgery involves the operative extirpation of tumor and all involved tissue obtaining clear margins (i.e remove any evidence of disease present). The vast majority of oral cavity cancers are treated with surgery initially. Early staged cancers, Stage I or II, can be treated with surgery alone. Depending on the location the surgery can be used with reconstructive options if the defect cannot be closed using simple techniques.

- **Radiation.** Radiation can be performed in three settings, definitive and (neo)adjuvant.
  - **Definitive Radiation (with or without chemotherapy).** This type of radiation treatment involves using radiation as the primary mode to treat the tumor. The goals of definitive radiation therapy is complete removal of all tumor with external sources of radiation. It is rare that this radiation is used in the definitive setting, and is usually used in the adjuvant setting.
  - **Adjuvant Radiation (with or without chemotherapy).** This refers to the use of radiation in combination with surgery. The goal of adjuvant radiation is to treat any remaining disease after surgical removal (e.g in circumstances with positive margins).
  - **Neoadjuvant Radiation (with or without chemotherapy).** Radiation given prior to surgery is referred to as neoadjuvant radiation. This is not routinely performed in oral cavity cancer, and is used in academic centers as part of larger studies.
- **Chemotherapy.** The use of systemic medications is used adjunctively with either surgery or radiation, and is used to target disease distant from the local site. It is not used as a primary treatment modality as it does not facilitate eradication at the primary site. Chemotherapy is often used in circumstances of advanced disease (Stage III or IV), or when certain risk factors for distant disease are present. Such risk factors include lymphnodes with disease that have extended out of their capsule (not contained), positive surgical margins, or involvement of nerves.
  - **Induction Chemotherapy.** This refers to chemotherapy performed prior to surgery or radiation. This may be used to see the biological response of the tumor to chemotherapy, as well as "shrink" tumors to a manageable size that can be better removed with surgery or radiation.
  - **Adjuvant Chemotherapy.** This refers to chemotherapy given after definitive treatment with another modality was performed (either surgery or radiation).
  - **Concurrent Chemotherapy.** This refers to the decision to administer chemotherapy and radiation concurrently after surgery. This may be the case in situations of predictors of aggressive disease on pathology.
- **Other Considerations.** Specific attention should be given to the presence or absence of neck disease in the patient. Oral cavity cancer has a higher percentage of occult disease (disease not present on imaging or physical examination). Part of the treatment algorithm is to determine if the neck should be treated.
  - **Therapeutic Neck Interventions.** If there is any presence of disease in the neck it should be addressed therapeutically. Positive neck disease is usually treated through surgical resection of the actual positive nodes, and all intervening nodes in the neck. This is to ensure accurate pathological characterization of the nodes in the neck, and

prevent recurrence in the neck (from missed disease). Definitive neck measures can also include definitive radiation to the neck.

- **Elective Neck Interventions.** In the absence of any clinical evidence of disease, an elective neck intervention may be performed. This means to treat the neck (with radiation or surgery) in circumstances that there is an "occult" or hidden disease that is not clinically apparent. Specific to oral cavity, all disease with primary (T-staging) greater than 2 (>T2), an elective treatment of the neck should be undertaken. In smaller T1 lesions (smaller than 2 cm), the decision to treat the neck is based on the depth of invasion. If the depth of invasion is beyond 4 mm, the risk of occult disease increases, and an elective neck dissection should be performed.

Prognosis. The prognosis and survival associated with oral cavity cancer is heavily influenced on the stage of the disease, the ability to safely remove the disease with clear margins, the ability to eradicate disease effectively within the neck, and the presence of aggressive pathological features. Patient centered factors also have been known to impact prognosis including presence of comorbid conditions, status of immune system, socioeconomic status, gender, and ethnicity.

- **Stage.** The factor with the highest impact on survival. Staging incorporates lymph node status, spread to local and vital tissues, as well as primary disease characteristics.

	Disease-Specific Survival at Five Years	Overall Survival at Five Years[1]
	Oral Cavity Cancer	Oral Cavity Cancer
Stage I	72%	59%
Stage II	58%	47%
Stage III	45%	36%
Stage IV	32%	27%

Oropharyngeal Cancer

Overview

The oropharynx is a term used to define the region bounded by the soft palate, the tonsils, the back of the throat, and the base of tongue. The different sites of involvement include the tonsils and its surrounding muscles (also referred to as the tonsillar pillars), the soft palate, the pharyngeal wall, and the base of tongue. Each site of the oropharynx may be approached separately with different guiding treatment principals.

Causes. Like all other head and neck cancers, chronic exposure to irritants such as alcohol tobacco is a significant risk factor for oropharyngeal cancer. However, in recent years, the impact of human papilloma virus (HPV) has been recognized as an ever increasing risk factor to oropharyngeal cancer. Patients with oropharyngeal cancer may have had no exposure to tobacco or alcohol. Other predisposing risk factors include male gender, family history, previous diagnosis of cancer in the head and neck, radiation exposure, as well as other environmental exposures.

Signs and Symptoms. Oropharyngeal cancers may present as later stages due to inadequacy in visualization, as well as nonspecific signs and symptoms. The majority of presenting symptoms center around the oropharynx's critical role in swallowing, breathing, and speaking.

- **Pain.** Frequently patients may present with throat soreness, that is non specific in quality and nature. Patients also present with ear pain. This is a type of "referred pain" whereby nerves in the oropharynx that communicate with the ear become irritated giving a false sensation that the ear is in pain. This is analogous to patients with heart attacks, having discomfort in their shoulders.
- **Masses.** The patient or other health care providers may notice a mass or lesion involving the throat, tonsils, or the back of the tongue.
- **Bleeding.** Bleeding from a site within the oropharynx may be a presenting sign. Any bleeding without full visualization chacterization of the involved site, warrants further workup.
- **Speaking and Swallowing Difficulties.** The presence of a tumor or lesion within the oropharynx times will impact a patients ability to speak or swallow. As lesions grow in size, patients may find it difficult to open their mouths (trismus), chew, or move their tongue. It is not uncommon to present with weight loss due to decreased oral intake. Tongue lesions may also impact a patients ability to properly articulate words.
- **Breathing Difficulties.** In advance cases in which the tumor has encroached on the upper airway, the patient may develop difficulty in breathing. This difficulty may be worsened in the declined position (e.g. when laying in bed).

- **Lump in the Neck.** Rarely cancers of the oropharynx can present as a single or multiple lumps in the neck. Persistence of neck mass beyond 1 month may warrant further work up.

Diagnosis and Workup. In addition to routine history and physical examination, the physician may perform ancillary tests and procedures in order to confirm the presence and type of oropharyngeal cancer, as well as to determine the presence of second primary cancers (SPC) or the spread of malignant disease elsewhere.

- **Biopsy.** Often times the first step in the diagnosis of oropharyngeal cancer is to perform a biopsy. Taking a biopsy will confirm the presence of abnormal cells under microscopic view, and is imperative in making the diagnosis of oropharyngeal cancer. Unique to oropharyngeal cancer is also the importance of determining the presence of human papilloma virus or Ebstein-Barr Virus (EBV) in tissue. This information helps guide therapy and counseling. Depending on the site of location, biopsy may be performed in different settings.
  - **In Office Biopsy.** If the lesion can be visualized (e.g. involving the soft palate), it may be determined that an in office biopy is the most efficient and effect method of obtaining tissue for analysis. This can be performed under local anesthesia with minimal discomfort to the pation.
  - **Operative Biopsy:** If the lesion has been visualized in a region of the oropharynx that is inaccessible (e.g. at the base of tongue) then an operative biopsy may be performed. This involves general anesthesia to gain direct visualization for tissue sampling. This is commonly known as a "direct laryngoscopy with biopsy".
  - **Lymph Node Biopsy.** If a patient presents with a neck mass, particularly in the setting of no identifiable lesion, the physician may sample tissue from lymph node. There are several types of lymph node biopsy.
    - *Fine Needle Biopsy (FNB).* If the mass can be felt by the clinician, then a small needle can be introduced with an attempt at extracting cells for microscopic assessment. The appearance of abnormal cells will help support the diagnosis of cancer. Sometimes, not enough cells are extracted, and repeat biopsies may need to be performed. This may also be performed with the help of ultrasound or computed tomography (CT) guidance
    - *Core Biopsy (CB).* Similar to the Fine Needle Biopsy, a core biopsy is performed by introducing a larger caliber needle, with extraction of tissue as opposed to cells. This core biopsy allows for extraction of more tissue and can be more useful, but often times not necessary, as an FNB is sufficient. This can

also be done with or without ultrasound or CT-guided assistance
- *Operative Biopsy.* If the location of the node is too deep, or not readily felt by a clinician, the surgeon may elect to perform biopsy under general anesthesia in an operating room.

- **Blood Work.** The physician may elect to perform routine blood analysis to assist in determining the presence of oropharyngeal cancer or other present diseases. Blood work may not be necessary, and the decision to obtain blood work is individualized to every patient.
  - **Liver Function Tests (LFTs):** Can be utilized to determine the presence of concurrent liver disease that may be associated with risk factors for the development of oropharyngeal cancer (alcohol consumption, hepatitis). Furthermore, abnormal values may indicate the presence of metastatic liver disease.
  - **Complete Blood Count (CBC):** This will identify the presence of any anemia that can sometimes be associated with poor nutrition, or chronic illness.
  - **Nutritional Blood Work:** If a patient seems nutritionally depleted, particularly in advanced cases, the clinician may elect to obtain laboratory work up to measure nutrition markers in the blood work. This may assist in determining if a patient requires supplemental nutrition.

- **Imaging.** Often times a physician may elect to obtain imaging that will help in better understanding the presence of cancer and any other underlying issues. Imaging may be performed of the primary site, or of the general region to better define disease extent. The physician may elect to obtain further imaging in situations in which they are concerned for local invasion (e.g. into bone, muscle, adjacent sites), or regional invasion (to the neck). Imaging is usually performed in the work up of oropharyngeal cancer, due to the location of lesions, and difficulty in defining the complete extent of tumor involvement.
  - **Chest X-rays:** Chest radiography may be obtained in order to define the presence of disease in the lungs. Often times patients with pharyngeal cancer, have a longstanding history of smoking, and may have associated lesions in their lungs that should be identified.
  - **Computed Tomography (CT):** CT-Scans usually provide a more detailed image of the head and neck region, identifying parts of the tumor that is not readily seen on exam, as well as the presence of regional disease not readily detected (e.g. in the neck). CT-Scans can be obtained with or without contrast. Given the complexity of the region, usually CT scans are obtained with scans, to help in identify the vascular architecture within the neck. However, this is not always necessary, and CT scans may be obtained without contrast in circumstances that preclude patient receiving contrast (iodine allergies, kidney disease). Paramount to guiding the treatment of

oropharyngeal cancer is precise mapping of the tumor to determine adjacent tissue involvement that cannot be assessed on routine clicical examination.

- o **Magnetic Resonanice Imaging (MRI):** MRI can also be utilized with or without contrast in order to provide superior visualization of soft tissue. Often times an MRI may be needed if there is indeterminante findings on other imaging modalities, with a need for more accurate mapping.
- o **18-Fluorodeoxyglucose Positron Emission Tomography (18-FDG PET):** FDG-PET scans may be performed with CT or MRI imaging modalities and are utilized for the identification of regional or distant metastases.
- o **Ultrasound (US):** Ultrasound may utilized to better characterize neck masses, or used in conjunction with biopsy techniques. US can indicate suspicious characters of lesions that would direct a physician to more aggressive workup (biopsy, excision).

Type of Cancer. The vast majority of cancers of the oropharynx are squamous cell carcinoma. However there are other cancers that also occur in this region that are on the differential diagnosis that must be considered.

- **Squamous Cell Carcinoma.** The vast majority of oropharyngeal cancers or squamous cell carcinoma. These cancers involve the malignant transformation of the mucosal lining within the oropharynx.
- **Salivary Gland Tumors.** The oropharynx houses small (minor) salivary glands that can be subject to malignant transformation. These cancers have a distinct behavior different from that of cancer involving the epithelial lining. They involve glandular tissue, with different treatment principles (*see Salivary Gland Cancer*).
- **Lymphoma.** Lymphoma may present as a lesion in the oropharynx due to the diffuse distribution of lymphoid tissue within the tonsils, pharynx, and base of tongue.
- **Mucosal Melanoma.** Melanoma, similar to the type of melanoma found in the skin, may also manifest in the oropharynx.
- **Soft Tissue Cancers.** Soft tissue cancers may present in the oropharynx, although rare. These involve sarcomas that may arise from muscle, fat, joint spaces.
- **Nerve Tumors.** Nerve tumors (e.g. neurofibroma) may also arise within the oropharynx.

Staging of Oropharyngeal Cancer. Once the appropriate diagnosis and work up of oropharyngeal cancer is complete cancer stage is determined. Currently, the method of staging used is the *American Joint Commission on Cancer (AJCC) Staging Manual* 7th edition.[1] The staging system is broadly referred to the TNM staging system, and is a descriptor of the factors that impact the staging of a cancer

- **Tumor Size (T):** This descriptor is used to categorize the size of the primary tumor.
    - **Tx:** Unable to assess primary tumor. This may be assigned in circumstances in which the primary tumor has not presented itself, but the patient has known lymph node disease
    - **Tis:** This refers to *carcinoma in-situ*, a type of cancer without invasion into the deeper structrues of the lining of the epithelial cells.
    - **T1:** The primary tumor is no greater than 2 cm.
    - **T2:** The primary tumor is between 2-4 cm in greatest dimension
    - **T3:** The pimary tumor is greater than 4 cm in greatest dimension.
    - **T4a:** Moderately advanced local disease. This is used to describe tumors with invasion into local tissues outside the confines of the oral cavity including: facial or cervical skin, the jaw, chin, muscle.
    - **T4b:** Very advanced local disease. This describes tumor that invades vital structures or spaces making eradiction of local disease difficult including: spaces around the muscles that assist in chewing, bones in the skull base, or involvement of the carotid artery (major blood supply to the brain).
- **Nodal Status (N):** This descriptor is used to describe the presence and number of lymph nodes in the neck.
    - **Nx:** Unable to assess nodal disease status.
    - **N0:** Absence of any nodal disease.
    - **N1:** There is one single node on the side of the tumor, no greater than 3 cm in its greatest dimension.
    - **N2a:** There is a single node 3-6 cm on the same side of the tumor.
    - **N2b:** There are multiple nodes on the same side of tumor, non greater than 6 cm in its greatest dimension.
    - **N2c:** Presence of any nodal disease opposite to the side of cancer, or both sides of the neck, but none greater than 6 cm in its greatest dimension.
    - **N3:** Presence of any nodes greater than 6 cm in greatest dimension.
- **Metastatic Disease Status (M):** This is used to describe the presence or absence of distant metastatic disease.
    - **M0:** No evidence of distant metastatic disease.
    - **M1:** Presence of distant metastatic disease.
- **Final Staging.** Once a value is assigned to each descriptor of the TNM cancer system, a final stage will be assigned.

Stage I	T1	N0	M0
Stage II	T2	N0	M0
	T3	N0	M0
Stage III	T1	N1	M0
	T2	N1	M0
	T3	N1	M0
Stage IVA	T4a	N0	M0
	T4a	N1	M0

T1	N2	M0
T2	N2	M0
T3	N2	M0
T4a	N2	M0

Stage IVB	T4b	Any N	M0
	Any T	N3	M0

Stage IVC	Any T	Any N	M1

- **Other Considerations.**
  - **Clinical Staging (cTNM):** The clinical stage refers to staging of the patient prior to treatment based on clinical information (physical exam, radiographic images etc).
  - **Pathological Staging (pTNM):** If surgical removal of tumor is performed, the pathologist will provide their own staging based on their microscopic and gross examination of all specimens.

Treatment Plan. Depending on the site of disease, the clinical staging, and patient factors (co-morbid health conditions, patient preferences) a patient specific treatment plan should be outlined. Broadly speaking there are 3 types of treatment that can be used in combination or separately depending on the type and stage of cancer. The decision to embark on a particular treatment plan should be made involving a multidisciplinary team of physicians (surgeons, radiation oncologists, and medical oncologists) and the patient. Patient specific goals and outcomes should be defined, with a thorough discussion of the risks, benefits, and alternatives of all the separate treatment types. Overall, there is no compelling evidence indicating any type of superiority of one treatment type over another. There are no valid studies comparing outcomes using the various modalities. This paucity in the literature highlights the very importance of effective communication between the patient and all providers.

- **Surgery.** Surgery involves the operative extirpation of tumor and all involved tissue obtaining clear margins (i.e remove any evidence of disease present as determined by microscopic analysis). Surgery is usually performed after the failure of other interventions (radiation with or without the use of chemotherapy). Primary surgical therapy can be considered for specific tumors of the oropharynx.
  - **Open Surgery.** Open surgery of the oropharynx is usually is limited by access to the region. Such surgeries require external access through incisions in the skin of the face and neck.
  - **Transoral Surgery.** Currently, ideal candidates for minimally invasive transoral surgeries of the oropharynx are being studied in clinical trials. Robotic and transoral laser surgeries may be an option in specific circumstances depending on patient and tumor factors. Transoral surgeries do not involve any incisions through the neck or face, with access obtained through the mouth.

- **Radiation.** Historically, radiation therapy has been the mainstay of treatment for lesions of the oropharynx. Radiation can be performed in three settings, definitive and (neo)adjuvant.
  - **Definitive Radiation (with or without chemotherapy).** This type of radiation treatment involves using radiation as the primary mode to treat the tumor. The goals of definitive radiation therapy is complete removal of all tumor with external sources of radiation.
  - **Adjuvant Radiation (with or without chemotherapy).** This refers to the use of radiation in combination with surgery. The goal of adjuvant radiation is to treat any remaining disease after surgical removal (e.g in circumstances with positive margins).
  - **Neoadjuvant Radiation (with or without chemotherapy).** Radiation given prior to surgery is referred to as neoadjuvant radiation. This is not routinely performed in the treatment of oropharyngeal cancers and is used in academic centers as part of larger studies.
- **Chemotherapy.** The use of systemic medications is used adjunctively with either surgery or radiation, and is used to target disease distant from the local site. It is not used as a primary treatment modality as it does not facilitate eradication at the primary site. Chemotherapy is often used in circumstances of advanced disease (Stage III or IV), or when certain risk factors for distant disease are present. Such risk factors include lymph nodes with disease that have extended out of their capsule (not contained), positive surgical margins, or involvement of nerves and blood vessels.
  - **Induction Chemotherapy.** This refers to chemotherapy performed prior to surgery or radiation. This may be used to determine the biological response of the tumor to chemotherapy, as well as "shrink" tumors to a manageable size that can be better removed with surgery or radiation.
  - **Adjuvant Chemotherapy.** This refers to chemotherapy given after definitive treatment with another modality was performed (either surgery or radiation).
  - **Concurrent Chemotherapy.** This refers to the decision to administer chemotherapy and radiation concurrently after surgery. This may be the case in situations of predictors of aggressive disease on pathology.
- **Other Considerations.** Specific attention should be given to the presence or absence of neck disease in the patient. Oropharyngeal cancer has a high rate of occult disease (disease not present on imaging or physical examination). Part of the treatment algorithm is to determine if the neck should be treated.
  - **Therapeutic Neck Interventions.** If there is any presence of disease within the neck the it should be addressed with a some type of therapeutic intervention. Positive neck disease is usually treated through surgical resection of the actual positive nodes, and all intervening nodes in the neck. This is to ensure accurate pathological characterization of the nodes in the neck, and prevent recurrence in

the neck (from missed disease). Definitive therapeutic intervention of the neck can also include radiation.
- o **Elective Neck Interventions.** In the absence of any clinical evidence of disease, an elective neck intervention may be performed. This means to treat the neck (with radiation or surgery) due to the potential for "occult" or hidden disease that is not clinically apparent. Elective neck interventions are usually performed for various sites of oropharyngeal cancer, and is dependent on the stage. Sometimes both sides of the neck should be treated if there is a high likelihood of occult disease bilaterally.

Prognosis. The prognosis and survival associated with oropharyngeal cancer is heavily influenced on the stage of the disease, the ability to safely remove the disease with clear margins, the ability to eradicate disease effectively within the neck, and the presence of aggressive pathological features.
- **Stage.** The factor with the highest impact on survival. Staging incorporates lymph node status, spread to local and vital tissues, as well as primary disease characteristics.
- **HPV.** The presence of human papilloma virus (HPV) seems to have a positive impact on tumor response to various treatment modalities, and continues to be studied.

	Estimated Disease-Specific Survival at Five Year[2] Oropharynx Cancer (1988-2001)	Estimated Disease-Specific Survival at Ten Year[2] Oropharynx Cancer (1988-2001)	Estimated Disease-Specific Survival at Five Year[2] Oropharynx Cancer (1998-1999)
Stage I	56%	42%	73%
Stage II	58%	46%	58%
Stage III	55%	44%	45%
Stage IV	43%	37%	32%

Nasopharyngeal Cancer

Overview

The nasopharynx is a term used to define the region bounded by the soft palate and the base of skull located in the back of the nose. Nasopharyngeal carcinoma is a rare cancer, and is predominantly found in Asian populations.

Causes. Like all other head and neck cancers, chronic exposure to irritants such as alcohol tobacco pose a significant risk for nasopharyngeal cancer. However, nasopharyngeal cancer is particularly associated with regions within Southeast China as well as other Asian areas. For reasons unknown (genetics, environmental exposure), individuals living or from these regions have a higher predisposition for developing cancer of the nasopharynx. Other risk factors include exposure to Ebstein-Barr Virus (EBV), environmental exposures (e.g formaldehyde), as well as foods prepared with nitrites (e.g dimethylnitrosamine).

Signs and Symptoms. Nasopharyngeal carcinoma (NPC) may present at later stages due to inadequacy in visualization, as well as nonspecific signs and symptoms.

- **Lump in the Neck.** Cancers in the nasopharynx most often present with a lump in their neck due to spread of the disease through lymphatics.
- **Headache.** Because the nasopharynx is close to the base of skull, carcinoma in the region may manifest itself as headaches.
- **Hearing Loss.** The nasopharynx is connected with both ears through the back of the throat. Often times, a mass in the nasopharynx will prevent drainage of fluid from the ear, causing decreased hearing, ringing, or ear infections.
- **Bleeding.** Bleeding from a site within the nasopharynx into the nose or mouth may be a presenting sign, and warrants further work up.
- **Swallowing Difficulties.** The presence of a tumor or lesion within the nasopharynx may prevent the patient from opening their mouth (trismus).
- **Nasal Congestion.** Because the nasopharynx is in the back of the nose, any masses or cancer in the area will make it difficult to breathe from your nose.
- **Neurological Problems.** The close proximity to the skull base, and potential to spread into the skull may cause neurological problems such as blurry vision, double vision, sensation loss/numbness, slurred speech, voice changes, or extremity weakness.

Diagnosis and Workup. In addition to routine history and physical examination, the physician may perform ancillary tests and procedures in order to confirm the presence and type of nasopharyngeal cancer, as well as to determine the presence of second primary cancers (SPC) or the spread of malignant disease elsewhere.

- **Biopsy.** Often times the first step in the diagnosis of nasopharyngeal cancer is to perform a biopsy. Taking a biopsy will confirm the presence of abnormal cells under microscopic view, and is imperative in making the diagnosis of nasopharyngeal cancer. Unique to nasopharyngeal cancer is also the importance of determining the presence of Ebstein-Barr Virus (EBV) in tissue. This information helps guide therapy and counseling. Depending on the site of location, biopsy may be performed in different settings.
    - **In Office Biopsy.** If the lesion can be visualized using a nasal camera, it may be determined that an in office biopsy is the most efficient and effective method of obtaining tissue for analysis. This can be performed under local anesthesia with minimal discomfort to the patient.
    - **Operative Biopsy:** If the lesion is small, or inaccessible in the a part of the nasopharynx that is difficult to reach under local anesthesia, it may be best to perform the biopsy in the operating room. This involves general anesthesia to gain direct visualization for tissue sampling. This is commonly known as a "direct laryngoscopy with biopsy".
    - **Lymph Node Biopsy.** If a patient presents with a neck mass, particularly in the setting of no identifiable lesion, the physician may sample tissue from lymph node. There are several types of lymph node biopsy.
        - *Fine Needle Biopsy (FNB).* If the mass can be felt by the clinician, then a small needle can be introduced with an attempt at extracting cells for microscopic assessment. The appearance of abnormal cells will help support the diagnosis of cancer. Sometimes, not enough cells are extracted, and repeat biopsies may need to be performed. This may also be performed with the help of ultrasound or computed tomography (CT) guidance
        - *Core Biopsy (CB).* Similar to the Fine Needle Biopsy, a core biopsy is performed by introducing a larger caliber needle, with extraction of tissue as opposed to cells. This core biopsy allows for extraction of more tissue and can be more useful, but often times not necessary, as an FNB is sufficient. This can also be done with or without ultrasound or CT-guided assistance
        - *Operative Biopsy.* If the location of the node is too deep, or not readily felt by a clinician, the surgeon may elect to perform biopsy under general anesthesia in an operating room.
- **Blood Work.** The physician may elect to perform routine blood analysis to assist in determining the presence of oropharyngeal cancer or other present diseases. Blood work may not be necessary, and the decision to obtain blood work is individualized to every patient.

- **Liver Function Tests (LFTs):** Can be utilized to determine the presence of concurrent liver disease that may be associated with risk factors for the development of oropharyngeal cancer (alcohol consumption, hepatitis). Furthermore, abnormal values may indicate the presence of metastatic liver disease.
- **Complete Blood Count (CBC):** This will identify the presence of any anemia that can sometimes be associated with poor nutrition, or chronic illness.
- **Nutritional Blood Work:** If a patient seems nutritionally depleted, particularly in advanced cases, the clinician may elect to obtain laboratory work up to measure nutrition markers in the blood work. This may assist in determining if a patient requires supplemental nutrition.
- **Epstein-Barr Virus (EBV):** This is a blood test that will determine exposure to EBV virus, as well as may correlate with disease burden. Studies indicate that treatment may be guided based on the EBV blood levels.

- **Imaging.** Often times a physician may elect to obtain imaging that will help in better understanding the presence of cancer and any other underlying issues. Imaging may be performed of the primary site, or of the general region to better define disease extent. The physician may elect to obtain further imaging in situations in which they are concerned for local invasion (e.g. into bone, muscle, adjacent sites), or regional invasion (to the neck). Imaging is routinely performed in the work up of nasopharyngeal cancer, due to the location of lesions, and difficulty in defining the complete extent of tumor involvement.
  - **Chest X-rays:** Chest radiography may be obtained in order to define the presence of disease in the lungs. Often times patients with pharyngeal cancer, have a longstanding history of smoking, and may have associated lesions in their lungs that should be identified.
  - **Computed Tomography (CT)**: CT-Scans usually provide a more detailed image of the head and neck region, identifying parts of the tumor that is not readily seen on exam, as well as the presence of regional disease not readily detected (e.g. in the neck). CT-Scans can be obtained with or without contrast. Given the complexity of the region, usually CT scans are obtained with scans, to help in identify the vascular architecture within the neck. However, this is not always necessary, and CT scans may be obtained without contrast in circumstances that preclude patient receiving contrast (iodine allergies, kidney disease). Paramount to guiding the treatment of nasopharyngeal cancer is precise mapping of the tumor to determine adjacent tissue and skull base involvement that cannot be assessed on routine clinical examination.
  - **Magnetic Resonanice Imaging (MRI):** MRI can also be utilized with or without contrast in order to provide superior visualization of soft tissue as well as the brain. Often times an MRI may be needed if there

is indeterminante findings on other imaging modalities, with a need for more accurate mapping.

- **18-Fluorodeoxyglucose Positron Emission Tomography (18-FDG PET):** FDG-PET scans may be performed with CT or MRI imaging modalities and are utilized for the identification of regional or distant metastases.
- **Ultrasound (US):** Ultrasound may be utilized to better characterize neck masses, or used in conjunction with biopsy techniques. US can indicate suspicious characters of lesions that would direct a physician to more aggressive workup (biopsy, excision).

Type of Cancer. The vast majority of cancers of the nasopharynx are squamous cell carcinoma. However there are other cancers that also occur in this region that are on the differential diagnosis that must be considered.

- **Squamous Cell Carcinoma (SCC).** The vast majority of nasopharyngeal cancers are squamous cell carcinoma. These cancers involve the malignant transformation of the mucosal lining within the nasopharynx. There are three types of SCC.
  - **WHO Type I (Keratinizing SCC).** These very similar to other head and neck SCC.
  - **WHO Type II (Nonkeratinizing SCC).** These are different from other SCC in appearance and behavior.
  - **WHO Type III (Undifferntiated or Poorly Differentiated SCC).** These are often found in younger patients with similar featrues to lymphoma.
- **Salivary Gland Tumors.** The nasopharynx houses small (minor) salivary glands that can be subject to malignant transformation. These cancers have a distinct behavior different from that of cancer involving the epithelial lining. They involve glandular tissue, with different treatment principles (*see Salivary Gland Cancer*).
- **Lymphoma.** Lymphoma may present as a lesion in the nasopharynx due to the diffuse distribution of lymphoid tissue.
- **Mucosal Melanoma.** Melanoma, similar to the type of melanoma found in the skin, may also manifest in the nasopharynx.
- **Soft Tissue Cancers.** Soft tissue cancers may present in the nasopharynx, although rare. These involve sarcomas that may arise from muscle, fat, ir joint spaces.
- **Nerve Tumors.** Nerve tumors (e.g. neurofibroma) may also arise within the nasopharynx.

Staging of Nasopharynx Cancer. Once the appropriate diagnosis and work up of nasopharyngeal cancer is complete cancer stage is determined. Currently, the method of staging used is the *American Joint Commission on Cancer (AJCC) Staging Manual* 7th edition.[1] The staging system is broadly referred to the TNM staging system, and is a descriptor of the factors that impact the staging of a cancer

- **Tumor Location (T):** This descriptor is used to categorize extent of tumor spread to surrounding regions.
    - **Tx**: Unable to assess primary tumor. This may be assigned in circumstances in which the primary tumor has not presented itself, but the patient has known lymph node disease
    - **T1:** The primary tumor is confined to the nasopharynx with minimal extension into nasal cavity or oropharynx (below).
    - **T2:** The primary tumor extends into the parapharyngeal space of the neck.
    - **T3:** The primary tumor has grown into bone of the skull base, or into the paranasal sinuses.
    - **T4:** the primary tumor has grown beyond the oropharynx into the hypopharynx, into the skull base with involvement of nerves, into the eyes, or into the infratemporal fossa or masticator spaces of the midface.
- **Nodal Status (N):** This descriptor is used to describe the presence and number of lymph nodes in the neck.
    - **Nx:** Unable to assess nodal disease status.
    - **N0:** Absence of any nodal disease.
    - **N1:** Lymph nodes confined to one side of the neck, all less than or equal to 6 cm in greatest dimension, above the supraclavicular fossa (the clavicle), and/or unilateral or bilateral retropharyngeal lymph nodes, less than or equal to 6 cm in greatest dimension
    - **N2:** Lymph node involvement on both sides of the neck, above the supraclavicular fossa, no greater than 6 cm in greatest dimension.
    - **N3a:** Any node greater than 6 cm in dimensions.
    - **N3b:** Any supraclavicular fossa nodes.
- **Metastatic Disease Status (M):** This is used to describe the presence or absence of distant metastatic disease.
    - **M0:** No evidence of distant metastatic disease.
    - **M1:** Presence of distant metastatic disease.
- **Final Staging.** Once a value is assigned to each descriptor of the TNM cancer system, a final stage will be assigned.

Stage 0	Tis	N0	M0
Stage 1	T1	N0	M0
Stage 2	T1	N1	M0
	T2	N0	M0
	T2	N1	M0
Stage 3	T1	N2	M0
	T2	N2	M0
	T3	N0	M0
	T3	N1	M0
	T3	N2	M0
Stage 4a	T4	N0	M0
	T4	N1	M0

	T4	N2	M0
Stage 4b	Any T	N3	M0
Stage 4c	Any T	Any N	M1

- **Other Considerations.**
  - **Clinical Staging (cTNM):** The clinical stage refers to staging of the patient prior to treatment based on clinical information (physical exam, radiographic images etc).
  - **Pathological Staging (pTNM):** If surgical removal of tumor is performed, the pathologist will provide their own staging based on their microscopic and gross examination of all specimens.

Treatment Plan. Depending on the site of disease, the clinical staging, and patient factors (co-morbid health conditions, patient preferences) a patient specific treatment plan should be outlined. Broadly speaking there are 3 types of treatment that can be used in combination or separately depending on the type and stage of cancer. The decision to embark on a particular treatment plan should be made involving a multidisciplinary team of physicians (surgeons, radiation oncologists, and medical oncologists) and the patient. Patient specific goals and outcomes should be defined, with a thorough discussion of the risks, benefits, and alternatives of all the separate treatment types. Broadly state, nasopharyngeal cancer is usually treated with Radiation with or without chemotherapy.

- **Surgery.** Surgery is usually limited to performing biopsies. . Definitive surgery is not usually preformed as a primary treatment modality. A surgeon may also elect to perform surgery in treatment of the neck (*see elective neck interventions and therapeutic neck interventions*).
- **Radiation.** Radiation therapy has been the mainstay of treatment for lesions of the nasopharynx.
  - **Definitive Radiation (with or without chemotherapy).** This type of radiation treatment involves using radiation as the primary mode to treat the tumor. The goals of definitive radiation therapy is complete removal of all tumor with external sources of radiation.
- **Chemotherapy.** The use of systemic medications is used adjunctively usually with radiation, and is used to target disease distant from the local site. It is not used as a primary treatment modality as it does not facilitate eradication at the primary site. Chemotherapy is often used in circumstances of advanced disease (Stage III or IV), or when certain risk factors for distant disease are present. Such risk factors include lymph nodes with disease that have extended out of their capsule (not contained), positive surgical margins, or involvement of nerves and blood vessels.
  - **Induction Chemotherapy.** This refers to chemotherapy performed prior to surgery or radiation. This may be used to determine the biological response of the tumor to chemotherapy, as well as "shrink" tumors to a manageable size that can be better removed with surgery or radiation.

- o **Adjuvant Chemotherapy.** This refers to chemotherapy given after definitive treatment with another modality was performed (usually radiation).
- **Other Considerations.** Specific attention should be given to the presence or absence of neck disease in the patient. Nasopharyngeal cancer has a high rate of occult disease (disease not present on imaging or physical examination). Treatment of both sides of the neck is usually done in addition to the primary site, regardless of whether disease is actually present.
  - o **Therapeutic Neck Interventions.** If there is any presence of disease within the neck it should be addressed with a some type of therapeutic intervention. Positive neck disease is usually treated through surgical resection or radiation of the actual positive nodes, and all intervening nodes in the neck. This is to ensure accurate pathological characterization of the nodes in the neck, and prevent recurrence in the neck (from missed disease).
  - o **Elective Neck Interventions.** In the absence of any clinical evidence of disease, an elective neck intervention should be performed. This means to treat the neck (with radiation or surgery) due to the potential for "occult" or hidden disease that is not clinically apparent. Elective neck interventions are usually performed for all nasopharyngeal cancers.

Prognosis. The prognosis and survival associated with nasopharyngeal cancer is heavily influenced on the stage of the disease, spread to surrounding structures, co-infection with EBV virus, as well as response to radiation and chemotherapy.

- **Stage.** The factor with the highest impact on survival. Staging incorporates lymph node status, spread to local and vital tissues, as well as primary disease characteristics.
- **EBV.** The presence of Ebstein-Barr Virus (EBV) seems to have a positive impact on tumor response to various treatment modalities, and continues to be studied.

	Estimated Disease-Specific Survival at Five Year[3]	Estimated Disease-Specific Survival at Ten Years[3]	Estimated Disease-Specific Survival at Five Year[4]
	Nasopharynx Cancer(1988-2001)	Nasopharynx Cancer(1988-2001)	Nasopharynx Cancer(1998-1999)
Stage I	72%	63%	72%
Stage II	64%	52%	64%
Stage III	62%	46%	62%
Stage IV	38%	37%	38%

Hypopharyngeal Cancer

Overview

The hypopharynx is the part of the throat beyond the oropharynx down to the level of the beginning of the esophagus. The hypopharynx has separate sites: lateral pharyngeal wall (the sides of the throat), posterior pharyngeal wall (back of the throat), postcricoid pharynx (before the esophagus), and the pyriform sinsues (the extension of the sides of the lateral walls).

Causes. Like all other head and neck cancers, chronic exposure to irritants such as alcohol and tobacco pose a significant risk to the development of hypopharyngeal cancer. Plummer-Vinson syndrome, characterized by iron deficiency anemia as well as swallowing problems, is also a risk factor for the development of hypopharyngeal cancer. Other risk factors include asbestos exposure, radiation exposure, or genetic or family predisposition to the development of cancer.

Signs and Symptoms. Hyopharyngeal carcinoma may present at later stages due to inadequacy in visualization, as well as nonspecific signs and symptoms.

- **Lump in the Neck.** Commonly nasopharyngeal cancers may present as persistent enlarged masses in the neck.
- **Pain.** Frequently patients may present with throat soreness, that is non specific in quality and nature. Patients also present with ear pain. This is a type of "referred pain" whereby nerves in the hypopharynx that communicate with the ear become irritated giving a false sensation that the ear is in pain. This is analogous to patients with heart attacks, having discomfort in their shoulders.
- **Bleeding.** Bleeding from a site within the hypopharynx may be a presenting sign. Any bleeding without full visualization or chacterization of the involved site, warrants further workup.
- **Speaking and Swallowing Difficulties.** The presence of a tumor or lesion within the hypopharynx often times will impact a patients ability to speak or swallow. Patients may have a hoarseness, or changes in voice quality. Patients may also develop a sensation of something in their throat (globus), or pain with swallowing.
- **Breathing Difficulties.** In advance cases in which the tumor has encroached on the upper airway, the patient may develop difficulty in breathing. This difficulty may be worsened in the declined position (e.g. when laying in bed).

Diagnosis and Workup. In addition to routine history and physical examination, the physician may perform ancillary tests and procedures in order to confirm the presence and type of hypopharyngeal cancer, as well as to determine the presence of second primary cancers (SPC) or the spread of malignant disease elsewhere.

- **Biopsy.** Often times the first step in the diagnosis of hypopharyngeal cancer is to perform a biopsy. Taking a biopsy will confirm the presence of abnormal cells under microscopic view, and is imperative in making the diagnosis of hypopharyngeal cancer.
    - **In Office Biopsy.** Although not routinely performed, it is possible to obtain tissue sample in the office using local anesthesia and endoscopic scopes. This however is not routinely performed due to difficulty in complete visualization.
    - **Operative Biopsy:** More routinely, hypopharyngeal biopsies are performed in the operating room under general anesthesia. This allows for more complete visualization and mapping of the tumor and tissue sampling, and is known as "direct laryngoscopy with biopsy".
    - **Lymph Node Biopsy.** If a patient presents with a neck mass, particularly in the setting of no identifiable lesion, the physician may sample tissue from lymph node. There are several types of lymph node biopsy.
        - *Fine Needle Biopsy (FNB).* If the mass can be felt by the clinician, then a small needle can be introduced with an attempt at extracting cells for microscopic assessment. The appearance of abnormal cells will help support the diagnosis of cancer. Sometimes, not enough cells are extracted, and repeat biopsies may need to be performed. This may also be performed with the help of ultrasound or computed tomography (CT) guidance
        - *Core Biopsy (CB).* Similar to the Fine Needle Biopsy, a core biopsy is performed by introducing a larger caliber needle, with extraction of tissue as opposed to cells. This core biopsy allows for extraction of more tissue and can be more useful, but often times not necessary, as an FNB is sufficient. This can also be done with or without ultrasound or CT-guided assistance
        - *Operative Biopsy.* If the location of the node is too deep, or not readily felt by a clinician, the surgeon may elect to perform biopsy under general anesthesia in an operating room.
- **Blood Work.** The physician may elect to perform routine blood analysis to assist in determining the presence of oropharyngeal cancer or other present diseases. Blood work may not be necessary, and the decision to obtain blood work is individualized to every patient.
    - **Liver Function Tests (LFTs):** Can be utilized to determine the presence of concurrent liver disease that may be associated with risk factors for the development of oropharyngeal cancer (alcohol consumption, hepatitis). Furthermore, abnormal values may indicate the presence of metastatic liver disease.

- **Complete Blood Count (CBC):** This will identify the presence of any anemia that can sometimes be associated with poor nutrition, or chronic illness.
- **Nutritional Blood Work:** If a patient seems nutritionally depleted, particularly in advanced cases, the clinician may elect to obtain laboratory work up to measure nutrition markers in the blood work. This may assist in determining if a patient requires supplemental nutrition.

- **Imaging.** Often times a physician may elect to obtain imaging that will help in better understanding the presence of cancer and any other underlying issues. Imaging may be performed of the primary site, or of the general region to better define disease extent. The physician may elect to obtain further imaging in situations in which they are concerned for local invasion (e.g. into bone, muscle, adjacent sites), or regional invasion (to the neck).
  - **Chest X-rays:** Chest radiography may be obtained in order to define the presence of disease in the lungs. Often times patients with pharyngeal cancer, have a longstanding history of smoking, and may have associated lesions in their lungs that should be identified.
  - **Computed Tomography (CT):** CT-Scans usually provide a more detailed image of the head and neck region, identifying parts of the tumor that is not readily seen on exam, as well as the presence of regional disease not readily detected (e.g. in the neck). CT-Scans can be obtained with or without contrast. Given the complexity of the region, usually CT scans are obtained with scans, to help in identify the vascular architecture within the neck. However, this is not always necessary, and CT scans may be obtained without contrast in circumstances that preclude patient receiving contrast (iodine allergies, kidney disease).
  - **Magnetic Resonanice Imaging (MRI):** MRI can also be utilized with or without contrast in order to provide superior visualization of soft tissue as well as the brain. Often times an MRI may be needed if there is indeterminante findings on other imaging modalities, with a need for more accurate mapping.
  - **18-Fluorodeoxyglucose Positron Emission Tomography (18-FDG PET):** FDG-PET scans may be performed with CT or MRI imaging modalities and are utilized for the identification of regional or distant metastases.
  - **Ultrasound (US):** Ultrasound may be utilized to better characterize neck masses, or used in conjunction with biopsy techniques. US can indicate suspicious characters of lesions that would direct a physician to more aggressive workup (biopsy, excision).

Type of Cancer. The vast majority of cancers of the hypopharynx are squamous cell carcinoma. However there are other cancers that also occur in this region that are on the differential diagnosis that must be considered.

- **Squamous Cell Carcinoma (SCC).** The vast majority of hypopharyngeal cancers are squamous cell carcinoma. These cancers involve the malignant transformation of the mucosal lining within the hypopharynx.
- **Salivary Gland Tumors.** The hypopharynx houses small (minor) salivary glands that can be subject to malignant transformation. These cancers have a distinct behavior different from that of cancer involving the epithelial lining. They involve glandular tissue, with different treatment principles (*see Salivary Gland Cancer).*
- **Lymphoma.** Lymphoma may present as a lesion in the hypopharynx due to the diffuse distribution of lymphoid tissue.
- **Mucosal Melanoma.** Melanoma, similar to the type of melanoma found in the skin, may also manifest in the hypopharynx.
- **Soft Tissue Cancers.** Soft tissue cancers may present in the hypopharynx, although rare. These involve sarcomas that may arise from muscle, fat, or joint spaces.
- **Nerve Tumors.** Nerve tumors (e.g. neurofibroma) may also arise within the hypopharynx.

Staging of Hypopharynx Cancer. Once the appropriate diagnosis and work up of nasopharyngeal cancer is complete cancer stage is determined. Currently, the method of staging used is the *American Joint Commission on Cancer (AJCC) Staging Manual* 7th edition.[1] The staging system is broadly referred to the TNM staging system, and is a descriptor of the factors that impact the staging of a cancer
- **Tumor (T):** This descriptor is used to categorize extent of tumor spread to surrounding regions.
  - **Tx:** Unable to assess primary tumor. This may be assigned in circumstances in which the primary tumor has not presented itself, but the patient has known lymph node disease
  - **T1:** The primary tumor is confined to a single subsite of the hypopharynx and is no greater than 2 cm in its greatest dimension
  - **T2:** The primary tumor extends into an adjacent subsite of the hypopharynx and is no greater than 4 cm in its greatest dimension.
  - **T3:** The primary tumor is greater than 4 cm in its greatest dimension, or involves the beginning of the esophagus, or has caused immobility of the vocal cords..
  - **T4a:** Moderately advanced local disease. The tumor has extended to involve cartilage of the neck, muscles of the neck, or the thyroid gland.
  - **T4b:** Very advanced local disease. This describes tumor that invades vital structures or spaces making irradiation of local disease difficult including: the lining of the spinal column (prevertebral fascia), the upper chest (mediastinum), or carotid arteries.
- **Nodal Status (N):** This descriptor is used to describe the presence and number of lymph nodes in the neck.
  - **Nx:** Unable to assess nodal disease status.
  - **N0:** Absence of any nodal disease.

- o **N1:** There is one single node on the side of the tumor, no greater than 3 cm in its greatest dimension.
  - o **N2a:** There is a single node 3-6 cm on the same side of the tumor.
  - o **N2b:** There are multiple nodes on the same side of tumor, non greater than 6 cm in its greatest dimension.
  - o **N2c:** Presence of any nodal disease opposite to the side of cancer, or both sides of the neck, but none greater than 6 cm in its greatest dimension.
  - o **N3:** Presence of any nodes greater than 6 cm in greatest dimension.
- **Metastatic Disease Status (M):** This is used to describe the presence or absence of distant metastatic disease.
  - o **M0:** No evidence of distant metastatic disease.
  - o **M1:** Presence of distant metastatic disease.
- **Final Staging.** Once a value is assigned to each descriptor of the TNM cancer system, a final stage will be assigned.

Stage I	T1	N0	M0
Stage II	T2	N0	M0
	T3	N0	M0
Stage III	T1	N1	M0
	T2	N1	M0
	T3	N1	M0
	T4a	N0	M0
	T4a	N1	M0
Stage IVA	T1	N2	M0
	T2	N2	M0
	T3	N2	M0
	T4a	N2	M0
Stage IVB	T4b	Any N	M0
	Any T	N3	M0
Stage IVC	Any T	Any N	M1

- **Other Considerations.**
  - o **Clinical Staging (cTNM):** The clinical stage refers to staging of the patient prior to treatment based on clinical information (physical exam, radiographic images etc).
  - o **Pathological Staging (pTNM):** If surgical removal of tumor is performed, the pathologist will provide their own staging based on their microscopic and gross examination of all specimens.

Treatment Plan. Depending on the site of disease, the clinical staging, and patient factors (co-morbid health conditions, patient preferences) a patient specific treatment plan should be outlined. Broadly speaking there are 3 types of treatment that can be used in combination or separately depending on the type and stage of cancer. The decision to embark on a particular treatment plan should be made involving a multidisciplinary team of physicians (surgeons, radiation oncologists, and medical oncologists) and the patient. Patient specific goals and outcomes should be defined, with a thorough discussion of the risks, benefits, and alternatives of all the separate treatment types. Broadly state, nasopharyngeal cancer is usually treated with Radiation with or without chemotherapy.

- **Surgery.** Surgery is commonly performed in the treatment of hypopharyngeal cancer. The extent and type of surgery is heavily influenced on the site of lesion, as well as patient's general health status.
  - **Partial Laryngopharyngectomy:** This type of surgery involves the surgical removal of part of the pharynx (throat), and the voice box. It is used in early staged lesions.
  - **Total Laryngopharyngectomy:** In advanced lesions with involvement of the voice box and surrounding structures, surgery may involve removal of the entire voice box and pharynx (throat), in order to fully remove all present disease.
  - **Transoral Surgery:** Currently, ideal candidates for minimally invasive transoral surgeries of the hypopharynx are being studied in clinical trials. Robotic and transoral laser surgeries may be an option in specific circumstances depending on patient and tumor factors. Transoral surgeries do not involve any incisions through the neck or face, with access obtained through the mouth.
- **Radiation.** Radiaiton is another option for treatment of hypopharyngeal cancer.
  - **Definitive Radiation (with or without chemotherapy).** This type of radiation treatment involves using radiation as the primary mode to treat the tumor. The goals of definitive radiation therapy is complete removal of all tumor with external sources of radiation.
  - **Adjuvant Radiation (with or without chemotherapy).** This refers to the use of radiation in combination with surgery. The goal of adjuvant radiation is to treat any remaining disease after surgical removal (e.g in circumstances with positive margins).
  - **Neoadjuvant Radiation (with or without chemotherapy).** Radiation given prior to surgery is referred to as neoadjuvant radiation. This is not routinely performed in the treatment of hypopharyngeal cancers and is used in academic centers as part of larger studies.
- **Chemotherapy.** The use of systemic medications is used adjunctively with either surgery or radiation, and is used to target disease distant from the local site. It is not used as a primary treatment modality as it does not facilitate eradication at the primary site. Chemotherapy is often used in circumstances of advanced disease (Stage III or IV), or when certain risk factors for distant disease are present. Such risk factors include lymph nodes with disease that have extended out of their capsule (not contained), positive surgical margins, or involvement of nerves and blood vessels.

- o **Induction Chemotherapy.** This refers to chemotherapy performed prior to surgery or radiation. This may be used to determine the biological response of the tumor to chemotherapy, as well as "shrink" tumors to a manageable size that can be better removed with surgery or radiation.
  - o **Adjuvant Chemotherapy.** This refers to chemotherapy given after definitive treatment with another modality was performed (either surgery or radiation).
  - o **Concurrent Chemotherapy.** This refers to the decision to administer chemotherapy and radiation concurrently after surgery. This may be the case in situations of predictors of aggressive disease on pathology.
- **Other Considerations.** Specific attention should be given to the presence or absence of neck disease in the patient. Hypopharyngeal cancer has a high rate of occult disease (disease not present on imaging or physical examination).
  - o **Therapeutic Neck Interventions.** If there is any presence of disease within the neck it should be addressed with some type of therapeutic intervention. Positive neck disease is usually treated through surgical resection or radiation of the actual positive nodes, and all intervening nodes in the neck. This is to ensure accurate pathological characterization of the nodes in the neck, and prevent recurrence in the neck (from missed disease).
  - o **Elective Neck Interventions.** In the absence of any clinical evidence of disease, an elective neck intervention should be performed. This means to treat the neck (with radiation or surgery) due to the potential for "occult" or hidden disease that is not clinically apparent.

Prognosis. The prognosis and survival associated with hypopharyngeal cancer is heavily influenced on the stage of the disease, spread to surrounding structures, as well as response to radiation and chemotherapy.

- **Stage.** The factor with the highest impact on survival. Staging incorporates lymph node status, spread to local and vital tissues, as well as primary disease characteristics.[4]

Estimated Disease-Specific Survival at Ten Years

Hypopharynx Cancer (1988-2001)

Stage I	27%
Stage II	25%
Stage III	19%
Stage IV	15%

Laryngeal Cancer

Overview

The larynx, also known as the voice box, is responsible for speaking, breathing, and protection of the lungs. It has three different subsites: supraglottis, glottis, and subglottis. The supraglottis is the region immediately above the vocal cords. The glottis is the region that includes the vocal cords. The subglottis is the region immediately below the vocal cords.

Causes. Like all other head and neck cancers, chronic exposure to irritants such as alcohol and tobacco pose a significant risk to the development of laryngeal cancer. Plummer-Vinson syndrome, characterized by iron deficiency anemia as well as swallowing problems, is also a risk factor for the development of laryngeal cancer cancer. Other risk factors include asbestos exposure, radiation exposure, marijuana use, or history of HPV papillomatous infections in childhood.

Signs and Symptoms. Laryngeal cancers often present with signs and symptoms related to the close proximity of the vocal cords and esophagus.

- **Lump in the Neck.** Laryngeal cancers may present as enlarged neck masses.
- **Pain.** Frequently patients may present with throat soreness, that is non-specific in quality and nature. Conversely, patients may present with increasing pain with swallowing.
- **Bleeding.** Bleeding from a site within the laryx may be a presenting sign. Any bleeding without full visualization or characterization of the involved site, warrants further workup.
- **Hoarseness.** Frequently, patients will present with hoarse voice, or changes in voice quality. Any voice changes that do not resolve beyond three months of conservative management should be evaluated by a specialist.
- **Breathing Difficulties.** Patient's may report breathing difficulties or noisy breathing, particularly when lesions increase in size and encroach on the airway.
- **Swallowing Difficulties.** Masses near or around the esophagus or vocal cords may cause intolerance to solid food that may progress to intolerance to liquid. Patients may also have a sensation of food being stuck in their throat that does not resolve with throat clearing (globus).

Diagnosis and Workup. In addition to routine history and physical examination, the physician may perform ancillary tests and procedures in order to confirm the presence and type of laryngeal cancer, as well as to determine the presence of second primary cancers (SPC) or the spread of malignant disease elsewhere.

- **Biopsy.** Often times the first step in the diagnosis of laryngeal cancer is to perform a biopsy. Taking a biopsy will confirm the presence of abnormal cells under microscopic view, and is imperative in making the diagnosis of laryngeal cancer.
  - **Operative Biopsy:** Laryngeal biopsies are performed in the operating room under general anesthesia. This allows for more complete visualization and mapping of the tumor and tissue sampling, and is known as "direct laryngoscopy with biopsy".
  - **Lymph Node Biopsy.** If a patient presents with a neck mass, particularly in the setting of no identifiable lesion, the physician may sample tissue from lymph node. There are several types of lymph node biopsy.
    - *Fine Needle Biopsy (FNB).* If the mass can be felt by the clinician, then a small needle can be introduced with an attempt at extracting cells for microscopic assessment. The appearance of abnormal cells will help support the diagnosis of cancer. Sometimes, not enough cells are extracted, and repeat biopsies may need to be performed. This may also be performed with the help of ultrasound or computed tomography (CT) guidance
    - *Core Biopsy (CB).* Similar to the Fine Needle Biopsy, a core biopsy is performed by introducing a larger caliber needle, with extraction of tissue as opposed to cells. This core biopsy allows for extraction of more tissue and can be more useful, but often times not necessary, as an FNB is sufficient. This can also be done with or without ultrasound or CT-guided assistance
    - *Operative Biopsy.* If the location of the node is too deep, or not readily felt by a clinician, the surgeon may elect to perform biopsy under general anesthesia in an operating room.
- **Blood Work.** The physician may elect to perform routine blood analysis to assist in determining the presence of oropharyngeal cancer or other present diseases. Blood work may not be necessary, and the decision to obtain blood work is individualized to every patient.
  - **Liver Function Tests (LFTs):** Can be utilized to determine the presence of concurrent liver disease that may be associated with risk factors for the development of oropharyngeal cancer (alcohol consumption, hepatitis). Furthermore, abnormal values may indicate the presence of metastatic liver disease.
  - **Complete Blood Count (CBC):** This will identify the presence of any anemia that can sometimes be associated with poor nutrition, or chronic illness.
  - **Nutritional Blood Work:** If a patient seems nutritionally depleted, particularly in advanced cases, the clinician may elect to obtain laboratory work up to measure nutrition markers in the blood work.

This may assist in determining if a patient requires supplemental nutrition.

- **Imaging.** Often times a physician may elect to obtain imaging that will help in better understanding the presence of cancer and any other underlying issues. Imaging may be performed of the primary site, or of the general region to better define disease extent. The physician may elect to obtain further imaging in situations in which they are concerned for local invasion (e.g. into bone, muscle, adjacent sites), or regional invasion (to the neck).
    - **Chest X-rays:** Chest radiography may be obtained in order to define the presence of disease in the lungs. Often times patients with larygneal cancer, have a longstanding history of smoking may have associated lesions in their lungs that should be identified.
    - **Computed Tomography (CT)**: CT-Scans usually provide a more detailed image of the head and neck region, identifying parts of the tumor that is not readily seen on exam, as well as the presence of regional disease not readily detected (e.g. in the neck). CT-Scans can be obtained with or without contrast. Given the complexity of the region, usually CT scans are obtained with scans, to help in identify the vascular architecture within the neck. However, this is not always necessary, and CT scans may be obtained without contrast in circumstances that preclude patient receiving contrast (iodine allergies, kidney disease).
    - **Magnetic Resonanice Imaging (MRI):** MRI can also be utilized with or without contrast in order to provide superior visualization of soft tissue as well as the brain. Often times an MRI may be needed if there is indeterminate findings on other imaging modalities, with a need for more accurate mapping.
    - **18-Fluorodeoxyglucose Positron Emission Tomography (18-FDG PET):** FDG-PET scans may be performed with CT or MRI imaging modalities and are utilized for the identification of regional or distant metastases.
    - **Ultrasound (US)**: Ultrasound may be utilized to better characterize neck masses, or used in conjunction with biopsy techniques. US can indicate suspicious characters of lesions that would direct a physician to more aggressive workup (biopsy, excision).
    - **Barium Swallow**: Swallow studies may be performed in order to determine the degree of obstruction, and presence of any other lesions within the esophagus.

Type of Cancer. The vast majority of cancers of the larynx are squamous cell carcinoma. However there are other cancers that also occur in this region that are on the differential diagnosis that must be considered.

- **Squamous Cell Carcinoma (SCC).** The vast majority of larynx cancers are squamous cell carcinoma. These cancers involve the malignant transformation of the mucosal lining within the larynx.

- **Salivary Gland Tumors.** The larynx houses small (minor) salivary glands that can be subject to malignant transformation. These cancers have a distinct behavior different from that of cancer involving the epithelial lining. They involve glandular tissue, with different treatment principles (*see Salivary Gland Cancer*).
- **Lymphoma.** Lymphoma may present as a lesion in the larynx due to the diffuse distribution of lymphoid tissue.
- **Mucosal Melanoma.** Melanoma, similar to the type of melanoma found in the skin, may also manifest in the laryx.
- **Soft Tissue Cancers.** Soft tissue cancers may present in the larynx, although rare. These involve sarcomas that may arise from muscle, fat, or joint spaces.
- **Nerve Tumors.** Nerve tumors (e.g. neurofibroma) may also arise within the larynx.

Staging of Laryngeal Cancer. Once the appropriate diagnosis and work up of nasopharyngeal cancer is complete cancer stage is determined. Currently, the method of staging used is the *American Joint Commission on Cancer (AJCC) Staging Manual* 7th edition.[1] The staging system is broadly referred to the TNM staging system, and is a descriptor of the factors that impact the staging of a cancer.

Supraglottis (T). The T staging will differ dependent on the site of the larynx that is Involved
- **Tumor (T):** This descriptor is used to categorize extent of tumor spread to surrounding regions.
  - **Tx**: Unable to assess primary tumor. This may be assigned in circumstances in which the primary tumor has not presented itself, but the patient has known lymph node disease
  - **T1:** The primary tumor is confined to a single subsite of the supraglottis with normal vocal cord mobility.
  - **T2:** The primary tumor extends into an adjacent subsite of the supraglottis (base of tongue, vallecula, true glottis), without any impact on vocal cord mobility.
  - **T3:** There is fixation or immobility of the vocal cords with or without invasion of the pre-epiglottic space or hypopharynx.
  - **T4a:** Moderately advanced local disease. The tumor has extended to involve cartilage of the neck, muscles of the neck, or the thyroid gland.
  - **T4b:** Very advanced local disease. This describes tumor that invades vital structures or spaces making irradiation of local disease difficult including: the lining of the spinal column (prevertebral fascia), the upper chest (mediastinum), or carotid arteries.

Glottis (T)
- **Tumor (T):** This descriptor is used to categorize extent of tumor spread to surrounding regions.

- **Tx:** Unable to assess primary tumor. This may be assigned in circumstances in which the primary tumor has not presented itself, but the patient has known lymph node disease
- **T1:** The primary tumor is confined to the vocal cords with normal mobility.
  - **T1a:** involving a single vocal cord
  - **T1b:** involvement of two vocal cords
- **T2:** The primary tumor extends into an adjacent subsite (subglottis or supraglottis), with or without vocal fold immobility.
- **T3:** There is fixation of the vocal cord with involvement outside the voice box (paraglottic space, or near adjacent cartilage)
- **T4a:** Moderately advanced local disease. The tumor has extended to involve the thyroid cartilage of the neck, muscles of the neck, or the thyroid gland.
- **T4b:** Very advanced local disease. This describes tumor that invades vital structures or spaces making irradiation of local disease difficult including: the lining of the spinal column (prevertebral fascia), the upper chest (mediastinum), or carotid arteries.

Subglottis (T)

- **Tumor (T):** This descriptor is used to categorize extent of tumor spread to surrounding regions.
  - **Tx:** Unable to assess primary tumor. This may be assigned in circumstances in which the primary tumor has not presented itself, but the patient has known lymph node disease
  - **T1:** The primary tumor is confined to only to the subglottis.
  - **T2:** The primary tumor extends up to the vocal cords with no impact on mobility.
  - **T3:** There is fixation or immobility of the vocal cords.
  - **T4a:** Moderately advanced local disease. The tumor has extended to involve cartilage of the neck, muscles of the neck, or the thyroid gland.
  - **T4b:** Very advanced local disease. This describes tumor that invades vital structures or spaces making irradiation of local disease difficult including: the lining of the spinal column (prevertebral fascia), the upper chest (mediastinum), or carotid arteries.

Nodal Staging. All nodal staging is the same for each laryngeal subsite.

- **Nodal Status (N):** This descriptor is used to describe the presence and number of lymph nodes in the neck.
  - **Nx:** Unable to assess nodal disease status.
  - **N0:** Absence of any nodal disease.
  - **N1:** There is one single node on the side of the tumor, no greater than 3 cm in its greatest dimension.
  - **N2a:** There is a single node 3-6 cm on the same side of the tumor.
  - **N2b:** There are multiple nodes on the same side of tumor, non greater than 6 cm in its greatest dimension.

- **N2c:** Presence of any nodal disease opposite to the side of cancer, or both sides of the neck, but none greater than 6 cm in its greatest dimension.
- **N3:** Presence of any nodes greater than 6 cm in greatest dimension.

Metastatic Staging. The M-staging is the same for all laryngeal subsites.

- **Metastatic Disease Status (M):** This is used to describe the presence or absence of distant metastatic disease.
  - **M0:** No evidence of distant metastatic disease.
  - **M1:** Presence of distant metastatic disease.
- **Final Staging.** Once a value is assigned to each descriptor of the TNM cancer system, a final stage will be assigned.

Stage I	T1	N0	M0
Stage II	T2	N0	M0
	T3	N0	M0
Stage III	T1	N1	M0
	T2	N1	M0
	T3	N1	M0
	T4a	N0	M0
	T4a	N1	M0
Stage IVA	T1	N2	M0
	T2	N2	M0
	T3	N2	M0
	T4a	N2	M0
Stage IVB	T4b	Any N	M0
	Any T	N3	M0
Stage IVC	Any T	Any N	M1

- **Other Considerations.**
  - **Clinical Staging (cTNM):** The clinical stage refers to staging of the patient prior to treatment based on clinical information (physical exam, radiographic images etc).
  - **Pathological Staging (pTNM):** If surgical removal of tumor is performed, the pathologist will provide their own staging based on their microscopic and gross examination of all specimens.

Treatment Plan. Depending on the site of disease, the clinical staging, and patient factors (co-morbid health conditions, patient preferences) a patient specific treatment plan should be outlined. Broadly speaking there are 3 types of treatment that can be used in combination or separately depending on the type and stage of cancer. The decision to embark on a particular treatment plan should be made involving a multidisciplinary team of physicians (surgeons, radiation oncologists, and medical oncologists) and the patient. Patient specific goals and outcomes should be defined, with a thorough discussion of the risks, benefits, and alternatives of all the separate treatment types. Broadly state, nasopharyngeal cancer is usually treated with Radiation with or without chemotherapy.

- **Surgery.** Surgery is commonly performed in the treatment of laryngeal cancer. The extent and type of surgery is heavily influenced on the site of lesion, as well as patient's general health status.
  - **Transoral Surgery:** Transoral surgery for laryngeal cancer can be performed with endoscopes and lasers. These minimally invasive procedures are used in specific circumstances whereby the tumor is confined, and can be fully visualized with a transoral approach..
  - **Conservation Laryngeal Surgery:** This type of open surgery involves the surgical removal of part of the larynx and the voice box. It is used in early staged lesions.
  - **Total Laryngectomy:** In advanced lesions with involvement of the voice box and surrounding structures, surgery may involve removal of the entire voice box in order to fully remove all present disease.
- **Radiation.** Radiation is another option for treatment of laryngeal cancer.
  - **Definitive Radiation (with or without chemotherapy).** This type of radiation treatment involves using radiation as the primary mode to treat the tumor. The goals of definitive radiation therapy is complete removal of all tumor with external sources of radiation.
  - **Adjuvant Radiation (with or without chemotherapy).** This refers to the use of radiation in combination with surgery. The goal of adjuvant radiation is to treat any remaining disease after surgical removal (e.g in circumstances with positive margins).
  - **Neoadjuvant Radiation (with or without chemotherapy).** Radiation given prior to surgery is referred to as neoadjuvant radiation. This is not routinely performed in the treatment of hypopharyngeal cancers and is used in academic centers as part of larger studies.
- **Chemotherapy.** The use of systemic medications is used adjunctively with either surgery or radiation, and is used to target disease distant from the local site. It is not used as a primary treatment modality as it does not facilitate eradication at the primary site. Chemotherapy is often used in circumstances of advanced disease (Stage III or IV), or when certain risk factors for distant disease are present. Such risk factors include lymph nodes with disease that have extended out of their capsule (not contained), positive surgical margins, or involvement of nerves and blood vessels.
  - **Induction Chemotherapy.** This refers to chemotherapy performed prior to surgery or radiation. This may be used to determine the biological response of the tumor to chemotherapy, as well as "shrink" tumors to a manageable size that can be better removed with surgery or radiation.
  - **Adjuvant Chemotherapy.** This refers to chemotherapy given after definitive treatment with another modality was performed (either surgery or radiation).

- o **Concurrent Chemotherapy.** This refers to the decision to administer chemotherapy and radiation concurrently after surgery. This may be the case in situations of predictors of aggressive disease on pathology.
- **Other Considerations.** Specific attention should be given to the presence or absence of neck disease in the patient.
  - o **Therapeutic Neck Interventions.** If there is any presence of disease within the neck it should be addressed with some type of therapeutic intervention. Positive neck disease is usually treated through surgical resection or radiation of the actual positive nodes, and all intervening nodes in the neck. This is to ensure accurate pathological characterization of the nodes in the neck, and prevent recurrence in the neck (from missed disease).
  - o **Elective Neck Interventions.** In the absence of any clinical evidence of disease, an elective neck intervention may be performed. This means to treat the neck (with radiation or surgery) due to the potential for "occult" or hidden disease that is not clinically apparent.

Prognosis. The prognosis and survival associated with laryngeal cancer is heavily influenced on the stage of the disease, spread to surrounding structures, as well as response to radiation and chemotherapy.

- **Stage.** The factor with the highest impact on survival. Staging incorporates lymph node status, spread to local and vital tissues, as well as primary disease characteristics.

	Estimated Disease-Specific Survival at Five Years[1]	Estimated Disease-Specific Survival at Ten Years[1]	Estimated Disease-Specific Survival at Five Years[1]	Estimated Disease-Specific Survival at Ten Years[1]	Estimated Disease-Specific Survival at Five Years[1]	Estimated Disease-Specific Survival at Ten Years[1]
	All Larynx Cancer(1988-2001)	All Larynx Cancer (1988-2001)	Glottic Larynx Cancer(1988-2001)	Glottic Larynx Cancer (1988-2001)	Supraglottic Larynx Cancer(1988-2001)	Supraglottic Larynx Cancer (1988-2001)
LocalizedNo spread into lymph nodes or other parts of body	83%	72%	90%	82%	64%	45%
RegionalSpread into neck lymph nodes	49%	35%	61%	47%	44%	30%
DistantSpread to distant part of body such as lungs, bone, brain, liver	19%	11%	34%	22%	15%	10%

Nasal and Sinus Cancer

Overview

The nose and sinuses that surround the nasal cavity may in rare circumstances develop cancer. The nasal cavity is defined by the area within the nose, excluding the skin; whereas the sinuses are collectively known as the paranasal sinuses and include: the maxillary sinuses, ethmoid sinuses, sphenoid sinuses, and the frontal sinuses. The sinuses are air filled pockets of bone that sometimes can harbor both malignant and benign tumors. Most often, growths within the nasal and paranasal sinuses are benign. However, the most common malignant tumor is squamous cell carcinoma, usually occurring in the maxillary sinus.

Causes. Nasal and sinus cancer are exceedingly rare, making it difficult to pinpoint the exact causes in most circumstances. As with other cancers of the head and neck, smoking seems to be a risk factor. Researchers also believe that genetic predisposition in addition to occupational exposures with nickel, chromium, leather, and wood workers may also contribute to the development of cancer in this region.

Signs and Symptoms. Sinonasal cancers frequently presents with symptoms related to their location within the nasal airway. However, the symptoms are often times non-specific, and may mimic other more common conditions. epistaxis, nasal obstruction, recurrent sinusitis, cranial neuropathy, sinus pain, facial paresthesia, proptosis, diplopia, or an asymptomatic neck mass.

- **Lump in the Neck.** Nasal and paranasal sinus cancers may sometimes present as a mass in the neck if the disease has already spread via lymphatics.
- **Nose Bleeds.** The presence of a tumor within the sinonasal tract may present as bleeding, particularly from one side
- **Sinus Problems.** Often times presence of a tumor may result in obstruction that causes infections, usually localizing to one side. Patients may also present with sinus pressure or headaches.
- **Vision Problems.** Due to the close proximity of the sinonasal tract to the eyes, patients may present with blurry or double vision.
- **Nasal Obstruction.** Patient's may report longstanding feelings of nasal congestion or change/loss of smell.
- **Neurological Problems.** Loss of facial sensation in regions of the face may occur if tumor has spread to involve nerves.
- **Lesions in the Mouth.** Cancers may extend into from the sinonasal tract and involve parts of the palate or mouth.

Diagnosis and Workup. In addition to routine history and physical examination, the physician may perform ancillary tests and procedures in order to confirm the presence and type of sinonasal cancer cancer, as well as to determine the presence of second primary cancers (SPC) or the spread of malignant disease elsewhere.

- **Biopsy.** Often times the first step in the diagnosis of sinonasal cancer is to perform a biopsy. Taking a biopsy will confirm the presence of abnormal cells under microscopic view, and is imperative in making the diagnosis of sinonasal cancer.
  - o **In Office Biopsy.** If the lesion can be visualized directly it may be determined that an in office biopsy is the most efficient and effective method of obtaining tissue for analysis. This can be performed under local anesthesia with minimal discomfort to the patient.
  - o **Operative Biopsy:** If the area to be biopsied is too difficult to access in the office a biopsy may be performed under general anesthesia in the operating room.
  - o **Lymph Node Biopsy.** If a patient presents with a neck mass, particularly in the setting of no identifiable lesion, the physician may sample tissue from lymph node. There are several types of lymph node biopsy.
    - ▪ *Fine Needle Biopsy (FNB).* If the mass can be felt by the clinician, then a small needle can be introduced with an attempt at extracting cells for microscopic assessment. The appearance of abnormal cells will help support the diagnosis of cancer. Sometimes, not enough cells are extracted, and repeat biopsies may need to be performed. This may also be performed with the help of ultrasound or computed tomography (CT) guidance
    - ▪ *Core Biopsy (CB).* Similar to the Fine Needle Biopsy, a core biopsy is performed by introducing a larger caliber needle, with extraction of tissue as opposed to cells. This core biopsy allows for extraction of more tissue and can be more useful, but often times not necessary, as an FNB is sufficient. This can also be done with or without ultrasound or CT-guided assistance
    - ▪ *Operative Biopsy.* If the location of the node is too deep, or not readily felt by a clinician, the surgeon may elect to perform biopsy under general anesthesia in an operating room.
- **Blood Work.** The physician may elect to perform routine blood analysis to assist in determining the presence of sinonasal cancer or other diseases. Blood work may not be necessary, and the decision to obtain blood work is individualized to every patient.
  - o **Liver Function Tests (LFTs):** Can be utilized to determine the presence of concurrent liver disease that may be associated with risk factors for the development of sinonasal cancer (alcohol consumption, hepatitis). Furthermore, abnormal values may indicate the presence of metastatic liver disease.

- o **Complete Blood Count (CBC):** This will identify the presence of any anemia that can sometimes be associated with poor nutrition, or chronic illness.
- o **Nutritional Blood Work:** If a patient seems nutritionally depleted, particularly in advanced cases, the clinician may elect to obtain laboratory work up to measure nutrition markers in the blood work. This may assist in determining if a patient requires supplemental nutrition.
- **Imaging.** Often times a physician may elect to obtain imaging that will help in better understanding the presence of cancer and any other underlying issues. Imaging may be performed of the primary site, or of the general region to better define disease extent. The physician may elect to obtain further imaging in situations in which they are concerned for local invasion (e.g. into bone, muscle, adjacent sites), or regional invasion (to the neck).
  - o **Chest X-rays:** Chest radiography may be obtained in order to define the presence of disease in the lungs. Often times patients with sinonasal cancer, have a longstanding history of smoking may have associated lesions in their lungs that should be identified.
  - o **Computed Tomography (CT)**: CT-Scans usually provide a more detailed image of the head and neck region, identifying parts of the tumor that is not readily seen on exam, as well as the presence of regional disease not readily detected (e.g. in the neck). CT-Scans can be obtained with or without contrast. Given the complexity of the region, usually CT scans are obtained with contrast, to help in identify the vascular architecture within the neck. However, this is not always necessary, and CT scans may be obtained without contrast in circumstances that preclude patient receiving contrast (iodine allergies, kidney disease).
  - o **Magnetic Resonance Imaging (MRI):** MRI can also be utilized with or without contrast in order to provide superior visualization of soft tissue as well as the brain. Often times an MRI may be needed if there is indeterminate findings on other imaging modalities, with a need for more accurate mapping. MRI can also assist in determining if there is involvement of nerves or the eye which is important in counseling patients regarding future directions of targeted therapies.
  - o **18-Fluorodeoxyglucose Positron Emission Tomography (18-FDG PET):** FDG-PET scans may be performed with CT or MRI imaging modalities and are utilized for the identification of regional or distant metastases.
  - o **Ultrasound (US)**: Ultrasound may be utilized to better characterize neck masses, or used in conjunction with biopsy techniques. US can indicate suspicious characters of lesions that would direct a physician to more aggressive workup (biopsy, excision).

Type of Cancer. Sinonasal tumors vary considerably from benign to malignant with treatment highly contingent on pathology, location, and extent of disease. It is important to recognize the different types of malignancies and their different behavioral patterns. The types of cancers can be categorized on the cells that they originate from. Epithelial based cancers come from the skin linining of the sinonasal cavities, whereas non-epithelial based cancers originate from soft tissue and bone.

- **Cancers of Epithelial origin.** Originate from the lining (or mucosa) of the sinonasal cavities
    - **Squamous Cell Carcinoma (SCC).** These are malignancies that originate from the skin lining inside the nose and sinus cavities. Behavior is highly dependent on the nature of the pathology.
    - **Salivary Gland Tumors.** Like other regions of the head and neck, minor salivary glands may give rise to cancers that have different degrees of aggression. (*see Salivary Gland Cancer*).
    - **Mucosal Melanoma.** Melanoma, similar to the type of melanoma found in the skin, may also manifest in the sinonasal cavities.
    - **Esthesioblastoma (olfactory neuroblasatoma).** This is a type of cancer that arises from the region of the nose that is responsible for smell detection.
    - **Sinonasal Undifferentiated Carcinoma.** This type of cancer is very aggressive. It is deemed "undifferentiated" because its cell of origin is unclear.
- **Cancers of Non-Epithelial origin.**
    - **Lymphoma.** Lymphoma may present as a lesion in the sinonasal cavity due to the diffuse distribution of lymphoid tissue.
    - **Soft Tissue Cancers.** Soft tissue cancers may present in the sinonasal cavity, although rare. These involve sarcomas that may arise from muscle, fat, or joint spaces.

Staging of Sinonasal Cancer. Once the appropriate diagnosis and work up of nasopharyngeal cancer is complete cancer stage is determined. Currently, the method of staging used is the *American Joint Commission on Cancer (AJCC) Staging Manual* 7th edition.[1] The staging system is broadly referred to the TNM staging system, and is a descriptor of the factors that impact the staging of a cancer.

Nasal Cavity and Ethmoid Sinus Cancer (T). The T staging will differ dependent on the site of the sinonasal cavity that is involved.
- **Tumor (T):** This descriptor is used to categorize extent of tumor spread to surrounding regions.
    - **Tx**: Unable to assess primary tumor. This may be assigned in circumstances in which the primary tumor has not presented itself, but the patient has known lymph node disease
    - **T1:** The primary tumor is confined to a single subsite with or without bony invasion.

- o **T2:** Tumor involves 2 subsites in a single region or extending to involve an adjacent region within the nasoethmoidal complex, with or without bony invasion
- o **T3:** Tumor extends to invade the medial wall or floor of the orbit, maxillary sinus, palate, or cribriform plate
- o **T4a:** Moderately advanced local disease. Tumor invades any of the following: anterior orbital contents, skin of nose or cheek, minimal extension to anterior cranial fossa, pterygoid plates, sphenoid or frontal sinuses
- o **T4b:** Very advanced local disease. Tumor invades any of the following: orbital apex, dura, brain, middle cranial fossa, cranial nerves other than (V2), nasopharynx, or clivus

Maxillary Sinus (T)

- **Tumor (T):** This descriptor is used to categorize extent of tumor spread to surrounding regions.
  - o **Tx:** Unable to assess primary tumor. This may be assigned in circumstances in which the primary tumor has not presented itself, but the patient has known lymph node disease
  - o **T1:** Tumor limited to maxillary sinus mucosa with no erosion or destruction of bone
  - o **T2:** Tumor causing bone erosion or destruction including extension into the hard palate and/or the middle of the nasal meatus, except extension to the posterior wall of maxillary sinus and pterygoid plates
  - o **T3:** Tumor invades any of the following: bone of the posterior wall of maxillary sinus, subcutaneous tissues, floor or medial wall of orbit, pterygoid fossa, ethmoid sinuses
  - o **T4a:** Moderately advanced local disease. Tumor invades anterior orbital contents, skin of cheek, pterygoid plates, infratemporal fossa, cribriform plate, sphenoid or frontal sinuses
  - o **T4b:** Very advanced local disease. Tumor invades any of the following: orbital apex, dura, brain, middle cranial fossa, cranial nerves other than maxillary division of trigeminal nerve (V2), nasopharynx, or clivus

- **Tumor (T):** This descriptor is used to categorize extent of tumor spread to surrounding regions.
  - o **Tx:** Unable to assess primary tumor. This may be assigned in circumstances in which the primary tumor has not presented itself, but the patient has known lymph node disease
  - o **T1:** The primary tumor is confined to only to the subglottis.
  - o **T2:** The primary tumor extends up to the vocal cords with no impact on mobility.
  - o **T3:** There is fixation or immobility of the vocal cords.
  - o **T4a:** Moderately advanced local disease. The tumor has extended to involve cartilage of the neck, muscles of the neck, or the thyroid gland.

- **T4b:** Very advanced local disease. This describes tumor that invades vital structures or spaces making irradiation of local disease difficult including: the lining of the spinal column (prevertebral fascia), the upper chest (mediastinum), or carotid arteries.

Nodal Staging. All nodal staging is the same for each nasal and sinus subsite.
- **Nodal Status (N):** This descriptor is used to describe the presence and number of lymph nodes in the neck.
  - **Nx:** Unable to assess nodal disease status.
  - **N0:** Absence of any nodal disease.
  - **N1:** There is one single node on the side of the tumor, no greater than 3 cm in its greatest dimension.
  - **N2a:** There is a single node 3-6 cm on the same side of the tumor.
  - **N2b:** There are multiple nodes on the same side of tumor, non greater than 6 cm in its greatest dimension.
  - **N2c:** Presence of any nodal disease opposite to the side of cancer, or both sides of the neck, but none greater than 6 cm in its greatest dimension.
  - **N3:** Presence of any nodes greater than 6 cm in greatest dimension.

Metastatic Staging. The M-staging is the same for all sinonasal subsites.
- **Metastatic Disease Status (M):** This is used to describe the presence or absence of distant metastatic disease.
  - **M0:** No evidence of distant metastatic disease.
  - **M1:** Presence of distant metastatic disease.
- **Final Staging.** Once a value is assigned to each descriptor of the TNM cancer system, a final stage will be assigned.

Stage I	T1	N0	M0
Stage II	T2	N0	M0
	T3	N0	M0
Stage III	T1	N1	M0
	T2	N1	M0
	T3	N1	M0
	T4a	N0	M0
	T4a	N1	M0
Stage IVA	T1	N2	M0
	T2	N2	M0
	T3	N2	M0
	T4a	N2	M0
Stage IVB	T4b	Any N	M0
	Any T	N3	M0
Stage IVC	Any T	Any N	M1

- **Other Considerations.**

- **Clinical Staging (cTNM):** The clinical stage refers to staging of the patient prior to treatment based on clinical information (physical exam, radiographic images etc).
- **Pathological Staging (pTNM):** If surgical removal of tumor is performed, the pathologist will provide their own staging based on their microscopic and gross examination of all specimens.
- **Esthesioneuroblastoma.** The staging of esthesioneuroblastoma is separate from other types of cancers.
    - Stage A: The tumor is limited to the nasal fossa.
    - Stage B: The tumor extends to the paranasal sinuses.
    - Stage C: The tumor extends beyond the paranasal sinuses.

Treatment Plan. Depending on the site of disease, the clinical staging, and patient factors (co-morbid health conditions, patient preferences) a patient specific treatment plan should be outlined. Tumours located within the maxiallary sinus, and nasal/ethmoid cavities may be managed differently. Furthermore, management of sinonasal malignancies further depends on the pathology, with different management protocols for squamous cell carcinoma, esthesioneuroblastoma, and mucosal melanoma. Broadly speaking there are 3 types of treatment that can be used in combination or separately depending on the type and stage of cancer. The decision to embark on a particular treatment plan should be made involving a multidisciplinary team of physicians (surgeons, radiation oncologists, and medical oncologists) and the patient.

- **Surgery.** Surgery may be performed in the treatment of sinonasal malignancies, with the extent and type of surgery guided by the location and degree of local invasion.
    - **Endoscopic.** Tumors limited in extent of local invasion and to certain subsites can be approached through the use of cameras and instruments introduced into the nose.
    - **Lateral Rhinotomy.** For larger lesions that extend further back in the nose that cannot be easily accessed through endoscopic approaches, may be approach by making an incision on the side of the nose.
    - **Anterior Maxillary Punch (Culdwel-Lac).** This approach involves entering the sinus through the mouth, drilling a hole into the front of the maxillary sinus.
    - **Craniofacial Resection.** For extensive lesions that are high in the nose or with extensive involvement of the skull base, a craniofacial resection may be performed.
- **Radiation.** Radiation is another option for treatment of sinonasal cancer.
    - **Definitive Radiation (with or without chemotherapy).** This type of radiation treatment involves using radiation as the primary mode to treat the tumor. The goals of definitive radiation therapy is complete removal of all tumor with external sources of radiation.

- **Adjuvant Radiation (with or without chemotherapy).** This refers to the use of radiation in combination with surgery. The goal of adjuvant radiation is to treat any remaining disease after surgical removal (e.g in circumstances with positive margins).
- **Chemotherapy.** The use of systemic medications is used adjunctively with either surgery or radiation, and is used to target disease distant from the local site. It is not used as a primary treatment modality as it does not facilitate eradication at the primary site. Chemotherapy is often used in circumstances of advanced disease (Stage III or IV), or when certain risk factors for distant disease are present. Such risk factors include lymph nodes with disease that have extended out of their capsule (not contained), positive surgical margins, or involvement of nerves and blood vessels.
  - **Induction Chemotherapy.** This refers to chemotherapy performed prior to surgery or radiation. This may be used to determine the biological response of the tumor to chemotherapy, as well as "shrink" tumors to a manageable size that can be better removed with surgery or radiation.
  - **Adjuvant Chemotherapy.** This refers to chemotherapy given after definitive treatment with another modality was performed (either surgery or radiation).
  - **Concurrent Chemotherapy.** This refers to the decision to administer chemotherapy and radiation concurrently after surgery. This may be the case in situations of predictors of aggressive disease on pathology.
- **Other Considerations.** Specific attention should be given to the presence or absence of neck disease in the patient.
  - **Therapeutic Neck Interventions.** If there is any presence of disease within the neck it should be addressed with some type of therapeutic intervention. Positive neck disease is usually treated through surgical resection or radiation of the actual positive nodes, and all intervening nodes in the neck. This is to ensure accurate pathological characterization of the nodes in the neck, and prevent recurrence in the neck (from missed disease).
  - **Elective Neck Interventions.** In the absence of any clinical evidence of disease, an elective neck intervention may be performed. This means to treat the neck (with radiation or surgery) due to the potential for "occult" or hidden disease that is not clinically apparent. If there is a high likelihood (>15%) of occult disease, an elective neck dissection may be performed.
  - **Orbital Involvement.** Involvement of the eye may necessitate surgical removal of the eye in order to fully eradicate the disease. This should be thoroughly discussed with the surgeon.

Prognosis. The prognosis and survival associated with laryngeal cancer is heavily influenced on the stage of the disease, spread to surrounding structures, as well as response to radiation and chemotherapy.

- **Stage.** The factor with the highest impact on survival. Staging incorporates lymph node status, spread to local and vital tissues, as well as primary disease characteristics.

Nasal Cavity.

	Estimated Disease-Specific Survival at Five Years[4]	Estimated Disease-Specific Survival at Ten Years[4]
Localized (confined to the primary site)	83%	77%
Regional (spread to nearby lymph nodes)	47%	38%
Distant (spread to another part of the body)	25%	22%

Paranasal Sinuses.

	Estimated Disease-Specific Survival at Five Years[4]	Estimated Disease-Specific Survival at Ten Years[4]
Squamous Cell Carcinoma	36%	31%
Adenoid Cystic Carcinoma	61%	45%
Adenocarcinoma	51%	46%
Other	48%	38%
Total	42%	35%

Skin Cancer

Overview

Cancers may arise within the head and neck, with an overall increase in rates seen across the United States and World Wide. Not all lesions are malignant, with many types of benign lesions that can arise from the skin of the face and scalp. In addition, certain lesions or growths may be considered pre-cursor lesions that need to be excised or observed.

Causes. The most significant risk factor for the development of a cutaneous lesion is exposure to both natural and artificial UV light (UV-A and UV-B). UV-B type light has been implicated more in causing cancer. The duration and intensity of exposure has been known to correlate with development of cancer. Patient related factors include skin type, with fairer skinned individuals having a greater affinity for developing skin cancer. Other patient related factors include history of radiation, presence of premalignant lesions, family history, previous scar or burn injury, being in an immunocompromised state, in addition to rare genetic syndromes.

Signs and Symptoms.

- **New or Changing Lesions.** The most common presentation of skin cancer in the head and neck is the appearance of a new lesion or change in previous lesion. Changes include increase in size, or development of ulcers or bleeding. A common mnemonic used for the evaluation of lesions is ABCDE.
    - **A-** Asymmetric lesions
    - **B-** Borders of the lesions are irregular
    - **C-** Color of the lesion is not consistent
    - **D-** Diameter of the lesion is greater then 5 mm
    - **E-** Evolving lesion size, shape, or color
- **Mass in Neck.** Certain types of cancer may present as a painless lump or mass in the neck, however this is not common.
- **Changes in Sensation.** Certain cancers may have an affinity to affect nerves of the face, head, and neck. Rarely, cancers may present as facial numbness or pain. Other cancers may cause the sensation of tingling in the affected region.

Diagnosis and Workup. In addition to routine history and physical examination, the physician may perform ancillary tests and procedures in order to confirm the presence of cancer.

- **Biopsy.** In order to accurately diagnose a tumor, the diagnosis must be confirmed on pathology.
    - **Biopsy.** The first step in the evaluation of a suspicious lesion is through biopsy.

- - **Excisional Biopsy.** This type of biopsy involves the removal of the entire lesion for analysis.
    - **Punch Biopsy.** This type of biopsy involves removal a portion of the lesion to evaluate its depth and pathological characteristics.
    - **Incisional Biopsy.** Although not commonly performed, this type of biopsy involves partial removal of a lesion for analysis.
- **Blood Work.** Blood work is not routinely performed in the work up of skin cancer. However, they may be performed in anticipation and part of a pre-operative workup prior to and operative biopsy.
- **Imaging.** Imaging is often times obtained after the diagnosis of cancer is confirmed on biopsy to assist in staging of the disease.
  - **Computed Tomography (CT)**: CT-Scans usually provide a more detailed image of the head and neck region, identifying parts of the tumor that is not readily seen on exam, as well as the presence of regional disease not readily detected (e.g. in the lymph nodes of the neck). CT-Scans can be obtained with or without contrast. Given the complexity of the region, usually CT scans are obtained with contrast, to help in identify the vascular architecture within the neck. However, this is not always necessary, and CT scans may be obtained without contrast in circumstances that preclude patient receiving contrast (iodine allergies, kidney disease).
  - **Magnetic Resonance Imaging (MRI)**: MRI can also be utilized with or without contrast in order to provide superior visualization of soft tissue that surrounds that surrounds the lesion. MRI may be helpful in distinguishing the tumor from surrounding tissue within the head and neck.
  - **18-Fluorodeoxyglucose Positron Emission Tomography (18-FDG PET)**: FDG-PET scans may be performed with CT or MRI imaging modalities and are utilized for the identification of regional or distant metastases.

Type of Cancer. There are two broad categories of skin cancers, melanomas and nonmelanoma skin cancer (NMSC).

- **Nonemelanoma Skin Cancers.**
  - Basal Cell Carcinoma (70-80% of all cancers)
  - Squamous Cell Carcinoma (15% of all cancers)
  - Merkel Cell Cancer (less than 1%)
  - Rare tumors arising from different skin components (e.g. hair follicles, sweat glands etc).
- **Melanoma**
  - About 5% of cancers
  -

Staging of Skin Cancers. Once the appropriate diagnosis and work up of the skin cancer is complete cancer stage is determined. Currently, the method of staging used is the *American Joint Commission on Cancer (AJCC) Staging Manual* 7th edition.[1] The staging system is broadly referred to the TNM staging system, and is a descriptor of the factors that impact the staging of a cancer. The staging will also be determined based on whether the lesion is a NMSC or melanoma.

Staging of Nonmelanoma Skin Cancer (NMSC)

Tumor mass (T). The T staging will characterizes the tumor itself.
- **Tx**: Unable to assess primary tumor. This may be assigned in circumstances in which the primary tumor has not presented itself, but the patient has known lymph node disease
- **T1:** The lesion is 2 centimeters or less in greatest dimension, and <2 high risk features*
- **T2:** The lesion is larger than 2 cm in greatest dimension, or tumor that is any size with > 2 high risk features*
- **T3:** The lesion invades cheek, jaw, or eye bones.
- **T4:** The lesion involves nerves of the base of the skull, or direct involvement of the axial or appendicular skeleton

*High Risk Features. These features may impact the staging because of their known correlation with worsening prognosis.
- **Depth of invasion.** If invades greater than 2 mm
- **Perineural invasion.** Invovlement of nerves.
- **Location.** Lesions involving the hair baring regions of the lip.
- **Pathology.** Poor appearance on pathology.

Nodal Status (N): This descriptor is used to describe the presence and number of lymph nodes in the neck.
- **Nx:** Unable to assess nodal disease status.
- **N0:** Absence of any nodal disease.
- **N1:** There is one single node on the side of the tumor, no greater than 3 cm in its greatest dimension.
- **N2a:** There is a single node 3-6 cm on the same side of the tumor.
- **N2b:** There are multiple nodes on the same side of tumor, non greater than 6 cm in its greatest dimension.
- **N2c:** Presence of any nodal disease opposite to the side of cancer, or both sides of the neck, but none greater than 6 cm in its greatest dimension.
- **N3:** Presence of any nodes greater than 6 cm in greatest dimension.

Metastatic Disease Status (M): This is used to describe the presence or absence of distant metastatic disease.
- **M0:** No evidence of distant metastatic disease.
- **M1:** Presence of distant metastatic disease.

Final Staging. Once a value is assigned to each descriptor of the TNM cancer system, a final stage will be assigned.

	T	N	M
Stage I	TI	N0	M0
Stage II	T2	N0	M0
Stage III	T3	N0	M0
	T1	N1	M0
	T2	N1	M0
	T3	N1	M0
Stage IV	T4	Any N	M0
	T4a	N1	M0
	T1	N2	M0
	T2	N2	M0
	T3	N2	M0
	Any T	Any N	M1

- **Other Considerations.**
  - ○ **Clinical Staging (cTNM):** The clinical stage refers to staging of the patient prior to treatment based on clinical information (physical exam, radiographic images etc).
  - ○ **Pathological Staging (pTNM):** If surgical removal of tumor is performed, the pathologist will provide their own staging based on their microscopic and gross examination of all specimens.

Staging of Melanoma Skin Cancer

Tumor mass (T). The T staging will characterizes the tumor itself and is heavily based on the depth of invasion within the skin.
- **Tx:** Unable to assess primary tumor. This may be assigned in circumstances in which the primary tumor has not presented itself, but the patient has known lymph node disease
- **T1:** The lesion is less than or equal to 1 mm in its greatest thickness
  - ○ **T1a.** No Ulceration
  - ○ **T1b.** Ulcer present
- **T2:** the lesion is greater than 1 mm but less than 2 mm in its greatest thickness
  - ○ **T2a.** No Ulceration
  - ○ **T2b.** Ulcer present
- **T3:** the lesion is greater than 2 mm but less than 4 mm in its greatest thickness
  - ○ **T3a.** No Ulceration
  - ○ **T3b.** Ulcer present
- **T4:** the lesion is greater than 4 mm in its greatest thickness
  - ○ **T4a.** No Ulceration

- ○ **T4b.** Ulcer present

Nodal Status (N): This descriptor is used to describe the presence and number of lymph nodes in the neck.
- **Nx:** Unable to assess nodal disease status.
- **N0:** Absence of any nodal disease.
- **N1:** There is one single node with disease in it
    - ○ **N1a.** Micrometastases.
    - ○ **N1b.** Macrometastases.
- **N2:** There is 2-3 nodes with disease in it
    - ○ **N2a.** Micrometastases.
    - ○ **N2b.** Macrometastases.
    - ○ **N2c.** In transit metastases, or satellite metastases
- **N3:** 4 or more nodes, nodes that are matted togehter

Metastatic Disease Status (M): This is used to describe the presence or absence of distant metastatic disease.
- **M0:** No evidence of distant metastatic disease.
- **M1a:** Presence of metastatic disease in distant skin or nodes
- **M1b:** Lung metastases, no liver involvement
- **M1c:** Any other organ involvement

Final Staging. Once a value is assigned to each descriptor of the TNM cancer system, a final stage will be assigned.

Stage IA	T1a	N0	M0
Stage IB	T1b-T2a	N0	M0
Stage IIA	T2b-3a	N0	M0
Stage IIB	T2b-4A	N0	M0
Stage IIC	T4B	N0	M0
Stage III	Any T	>N0	M0
Stage IV	Any T	Any N	M1

- **Other Considerations.**
    - ○ **Clinical Staging (cTNM):** The clinical stage refers to staging of the patient prior to treatment based on clinical information (physical exam, radiographic images etc).
    - ○ **Pathological Staging (pTNM):** If surgical removal of tumor is performed, the pathologist will provide their own staging based on their microscopic and gross examination of all specimens.

Treatment Plan. Depending on the site of disease, the clinical staging, and patient factors (co-morbid health conditions, patient preferences) a patient specific treatment plan should be outlined.

- **Surgery.** Surgery is usually the treatment option of choice for all stages of skin cancer.
    - **Nonmelanoma Skin Cancer.** Surgery typically involves removal of the lesion. Sometimes a neck dissection must be performed if there exists a high risk of microscopic disease within the nodes or parotid gland.
    - **Melanoma Skin Cancer.** Surgery also involves removal of the skin. If there is a high risk of involvement of the surrounding lymph nodes, a neck dissection may also be performed.
- **Radiation.** Radiation is often times indicated.
    - **Nonmelanoma Skin Cancer.** If the lesion is high risk with neural involvement, lymphatic or parotid involvement, bone involvement, or is a recurrent lesion then radiation may be administered after surgery.
    - **Melanoma.** Radiation is not usually administered in the routine treatment of melanoma skin cancer, however ongoing studies are looking further into this.
- **Chemotherapy.** Chemotherapy is not usually used in the treatment of skin cancers.
- **Interferon Therapy.** The FDA has approved the use of interferon in the treatment of Stage III melanoma skin cancer, with current ongoing studies identifying the exact role.

Prognosis. The prognosis and survival associated with skin cancer is heavily influenced on the stage of the disease, spread to surrounding structures, as well as response to therapy.

Salivary Gland Malignancies

Overview

Malignancies may occasionally arise from salivary glands located throughout the head and neck. There are major and minor salivary glands depending on their size and location. The major salivary glands are the paired parotid, submandibular, and sublingual glands. Minor salivary glands are smaller glands located within the lining of the mouth, nose, sinuses, and throat. Malignant or benign tumors may arise in any of the major or minor salivary glands. Other conditions may also present similar to tumors, and these include other non-malignant conditions such as acute or chronic infections, manifestations of other systemic illnesses, or salivary gland stones.

Causes. There is little understanding to the causes of salivary gland malignancies. Radiation exposure (treatment and environmental) has been linked to the development of salivary cancers. However, unlike other cancers of the head and neck, smoking and alcohol do not seem to be causative factors. Smoking does however seem to be related to the development of Warthin's Tumor, a benign tumor.

Signs and Symptoms. The signs and symptoms of salivary gland tumors is highly variable and dependent on the location.

- **Mass.** The most common symptom is the development of a painless mass either in the face, mouth, nose, or throat. These masses may be slow growing, or may increase in size rapidly. Masses in close proximity to the airway may grow to cause airway obstruction and difficulty in breathing.
- **Facial Numbness or Weakness.** Tumors that involve the nerves of the face may present with paralysis or numbness on the affected side.
- **Sinus Problems.** Salivary gland tumors that involve the sinonasal passageway may present with nasal obstruction, sinus infections, nose bleeds, or facial pressure.
- **Swallowing problems.** Lesions in the throat may also enlarge to cause difficulty in swallowing.

Diagnosis and Workup. In addition to routine history and physical examination, the physician may perform ancillary tests and procedures in order to confirm the presence of salivary gland cancer.

- **Biopsy.** In order to accurately diagnose a tumor, the diagnosis must be confirmed on pathology.
  - **Operative Biopsy/Definitive Removal:** The majority of salivary gland tumors are benign, and often time an operative biopsy is the first and only step required in its management. The gland or tumor

can be removed in the operating room under general anesthesia. This will provide tissue for analysis, as well as be therapeutic in removing the tumor.

- **Fine Needle Biopsy (FNB**). If the mass can be felt by the clinician, then a small needle can be introduced with an attempt at extracting cells for microscopic assessment. The appearance of abnormal cells will help support the diagnosis of cancer. It is not necessary to perform an FNB, and not all surgeons elect to do so. However, it may provide valuable information that will guide definitive operative biopsy.

- **Blood Work.** Blood work is not routinely performed in the work up of salivary gland malignancies. However, they may be performed in anticipation and part of a pre-operative workup prior to the operative biopsy.

- **Imaging.** Often times a physician may elect to obtain imaging that will help in better understanding the presence of cancer and any other underlying issues. Imaging may be performed of the primary site, or of the general region to better define disease extent. The physician may elect to obtain further imaging in situations in which they are concerned for local invasion (e.g. into bone, muscle, adjacent sites), or regional invasion (to the neck). Imaging may assist in determining if the tumor appears benign in nature, or has characteristics of a malignancy.

  - **Computed Tomography (CT)**: CT-Scans usually provide a more detailed image of the head and neck region, identifying parts of the tumor that is not readily seen on exam, as well as the presence of regional disease not readily detected (e.g. in the neck). CT-Scans can be obtained with or without contrast. Given the complexity of the region, usually CT scans are obtained with contrast, to help in identify the vascular architecture within the neck. However, this is not always necessary, and CT scans may be obtained without contrast in circumstances that preclude patient receiving contrast (iodine allergies, kidney disease).

  - **Magnetic Resonance Imaging (MRI):** MRI can also be utilized with or without contrast in order to provide superior visualization of soft soft tissue that surrounds that salivary glands. MRI may be helpful in distinguishing the tumor from surrounding tissue within the head and neck, as well as demonstrate characteristic features that assist in determining its likelihood of being malignant.

  - **18-Fluorodeoxyglucose Positron Emission Tomography (18-FDG PET):** FDG-PET scans may be performed with CT or MRI imaging modalities and are utilized for the identification of regional or distant metastases.

  - **Ultrasound (US)**: In some studies, ultrasound imaging has been used better characterize the salivary gland tumor and stratify the likelihood of malignancy. They also may be used to assist in guiding FNA biopsies.

Type of Cancer. Because of the complexity and varying types of cells with the salivary glands, tumors are diverse with varying degrees of behavior from benign to aggressive. The likelihood of malignancy varies on the location and type of gland that has developed.

- **Cancers of Epithelial origin.**
  - Mucoepidermoid carcinoma
    Adenoid cystic carcinoma
    Acinic cell carcinoma
    Adenocarcinoma, NOS
    Carcinoma ex pleomorphic adenoma
    Squamous cell carcinoma
    Polymorphous low-grade
    Adenocarcinoma
    Epithelial-myoepithelial carcinoma
    Clear cell carcinoma, NOS
    Basal cell adenocarcinoma
    Sebaceous carcinoma
    Sebaceous lymphadenocarcinoma
    Cystadenocarcinoma
    Low-grade cribriform
    Mucinous adenocarcinoma
    Oncocytic carcinoma
    Salivary duct carcinoma
    Myoepithelial carcinoma
    Carcinosarcoma
    Metastasizing pleomorphic adenoma
    Small cell carcinoma
    Large cell carcinoma
    Lymphoepithelial carcinoma
    Sialoblastoma
- **Tumors arising from blood and lymphatic vessles.**
  - Lymphoma
  - Hemangioma
- **Soft Tissue Tumors**
  - Haemangiopericytoma
    Malignant schwannoma
    Fibrosarcoma
    Malignant fibrous histiocytoma
    Rhabdomyosarcoma
    Angiosarcoma
    Synovial sarcoma
    Kaposi sarcoma
    Leiomyosarcoma

Liposarcoma
Alveolar soft part sarcoma
Epithelioid sarcoma
Extraosseous chondrosarcoma
Osteosarcoma
Malignant haemangioendothelioma

- **Metastatic Tumors.** Tumors from other parts of the body may manifest as metastatic disease in the salivary glands.

Staging of Salivary Gland Tumors. Once the appropriate diagnosis and work up of salivary gland cancer is complete cancer stage is determined. Currently, the method of staging used is the *American Joint Commission on Cancer (AJCC) Staging Manual* 7th edition.[1] The staging system is broadly referred to the TNM staging system, and is a descriptor of the factors that impact the staging of a cancer.

Tumor mass (T). The T staging will characterizes the tumor itself.
- **Tx**: Unable to assess primary tumor. This may be assigned in circumstances in which the primary tumor has not presented itself, but the patient has known lymph node disease
- **T1:** The tumor is 2 centimeters or less in greatest dimension, and does not grow outside the gland.
- **T2:** The tumor is larger than 2 cm in greatest dimension, but no greater than 4 cm, without evidence of growth outside the gland itself.
- **T3:** The gland is greater than 4 cm, or it has grown outside the gland itself.
- **T4a:** Moderately advanced local disease. Tumor invades any of the following: skin, jaw, ear canal, or the nerve that controls facial movement.
- **T4b:** Very advanced local disease. Tumor invades any of the following: base of skull, the pterygoid plates, and/or encases the carotid artery.

Nodal Status (N): This descriptor is used to describe the presence and number of lymph nodes in the neck.
- **Nx:** Unable to assess nodal disease status.
- **N0:** Absence of any nodal disease.
- **N1:** There is one single node on the side of the tumor, no greater than 3 cm in its greatest dimension.
- **N2a:** There is a single node 3-6 cm on the same side of the tumor.
- **N2b:** There are multiple nodes on the same side of tumor, non greater than 6 cm in its greatest dimension.
- **N2c:** Presence of any nodal disease opposite to the side of cancer, or both sides of the neck, but none greater than 6 cm in its greatest dimension.
- **N3:** Presence of any nodes greater than 6 cm in greatest dimension.

Metastatic Disease Status (M): This is used to describe the presence or absence of distant metastatic disease.
- **M0:** No evidence of distant metastatic disease.

- **M1:** Presence of distant metastatic disease.

Final Staging. Once a value is assigned to each descriptor of the TNM cancer system, a final stage will be assigned.

Stage I	TI	N0	M0
Stage II	T2	N0	M0
Stage III	T3	N0	M0
	T1	N1	M0
	T2	N1	M0
	T3	N1	M0
Stage IVA	T4a	N0	M0
	T4a	N1	M0
	T1	N2	M0
	T2	N2	M0
	T3	N2	M0
	T4a	N2	M0
Stage IVB	T4b	AnyN	M0
	AnyT	N3	M0
Stage IVC	AnyT	AnyN	M1

- **Other Considerations.**
  - **Clinical Staging (cTNM):** The clinical stage refers to staging of the patient prior to treatment based on clinical information (physical exam, radiographic images etc).
  - **Pathological Staging (pTNM):** If surgical removal of tumor is performed, the pathologist will provide their own staging based on their microscopic and gross examination of all specimens.

Treatment Plan. Depending on the site of disease, the clinical staging, and patient factors (co-morbid health conditions, patient preferences) a patient specific treatment plan should be outlined.
- **Surgery.** Surgery is usually the treatment option of choice for all stages of salivary gland malignancies (except T4b).
- **Radiation.** Radiation is often times given as part of the treatment of late stage tumors following surgery, or tumors that are not candidates for surgical resection (T4b).
  - **Definitive Radiation.** This type of radiation treatment involves using radiation as the primary mode to treat the tumor. Definitive radiation is usually reserved for T4b tumors.
  - **Adjuvant Radiation.** This refers to the use of radiation in combination with surgery. The goal of adjuvant radiation is to treat any remaining disease after surgical removal (e.g in circumstances with positive margins).

- **Chemotherapy.** Chemotherapy is not usually used in the treatment of salivary gland tumors. However, specific circumstances may warrant its use: spread of cancer beyond the head and neck, or when certain risk factors for distant disease are present: lymph nodes with disease that have extended out of their capsule (not contained), positive surgical margins, or involvement of nerves and blood vessels.
- **Other Considerations.** Specific attention should be given to the presence or absence of neck disease in the patient.
  - **Therapeutic Neck Interventions.** If there is any presence of disease within the neck it should be addressed with some type of therapeutic intervention. Positive neck disease is usually treated through surgical resection of the actual positive nodes, and all intervening nodes in the neck.
  - **Elective Neck Interventions.** In the absence of any clinical evidence of disease, an elective neck intervention may be performed. This means to treat the neck (with radiation or surgery) due to the potential for "occult" or hidden disease that is not clinically apparent. If there is a high likelihood (>15%) of occult disease, an elective neck dissection may be performed. However, these type of interventions are not routinely performed in the treatment of salivary gland tumors.

Prognosis. The prognosis and survival associated with salivary cancer is heavily influenced on the stage of the disease, spread to surrounding structures, as well as response to radiation and chemotherapy.
- **Stage.** The factor with the highest impact on survival. Staging incorporates lymph node status, spread to local and vital tissues, as well as primary disease characteristics.
- **Grade.** The histological grade has impact on prognosis.
- **Pathology.** The type of salivary gland tumor is also important in determining how aggressive it is, with impact on survival.
- **Site.** Major salivary gland tumors are more likely to be benign then minor salivary gland tumors, with better outcomes.

	Estimated Disease-Specific Survival at Five Years[4] Salivary Gland Cancer	Estimated Disease-Specific Survival at 10 Years Salivary Gland Cancer[4]
Stage I	96%	92%
Stage II	77%	67%
Stage III	73%	58%
Stage IV	37%	28%

	Estimated Disease-Specific Survival at Five Years[4] Salivary Gland Cancer	Estimated Disease-Specific Survival at 10 Years[4] Salivary Gland Cancer
Grade I	70%	57%

Grade II	60%	47%
Stage III-IV	39%	29%

	Estimated Disease-Specific Survival at Five Years Salivary Gland Cancer[4]	Estimated Disease-Specific Survival at 10 Years Salivary Gland Cancer[4]
Squamous Cell Carcinoma	46%	37%
Adenocarcinoma	60%	49%
Adenoid Cystic Carcinoma	84%	71%
Mucoepidermoid Carcinoma, Poorly Differentiated	90%	85%
Acinic Cell Carcinoma	96%	94%
Mucoepidermoid Carcinoma (Other)	96%	94%
Carcinoma in Pleomorphic Adenoma (Malignant Mixed Tumor)	82%	71%
Mucoepidermoid Carcinoma, Well Differentiated	99%	99%

	Estimated Disease-Specific Survival at Five Years	Estimated Disease-Specific Survival at 10 Years (minor salivary gland cancer)[5]	Estimated Disease-Specific Survival at 10 Years (adenoid cystic carcinoma)[6]
	Salivary Gland Cancer (all sites)*	Minor Salivary Gland Cancers	Adenoid Cystic Carcinoma
		1966-1991	1966-1991
Stage I	77%	83%	75%
Stage II	58%	53%	43%
Stage III	51%	35%	15%
Stage IV	30%	24%	15%

Thyroid Cancer

Overview

The thyroid is a butterfly shaped gland that sits in the neck in front of the trachea. It is involved in the regulation of metabolic activity of the body with physiological effects on sleeping, weight changes, energy, blood pressure, and heart rate. Like other glands throughout the body, the thyroid may be subject to malignant changes. There are four major types of thyroid cancer, papillary, follicular, medullary, and anaplastic.

Causes. Thyroid cancers may be caused by exposure to radiation (environmental, or as part of treatment), particularly as a child. There are other types of genetic conditions that also may be associated with thyroid cancers: familial medullary thyroid cancer, multiple endocrine neoplasia (MEN) type 2A and type 2B.

Signs and Symptoms.

- **Nodules.** Most often thyroid cancers manifest as single, painless nodules detected on routine physical exam, or as incidental imaging findings found for work up of other conditions.
- **Changes in Voice.** Rarely, in advanced cases thyroid cancers may cause hoarseness or changes in voice quality.
- **Swallowing Difficulties.** In advanced cases larger or aggressive tumors may impact a patients ability to swallow.
- **Breathing Difficulties.** In rare instances, tumor growth may impact patient breathing.

Diagnosis and Workup. In addition to routine history and physical examination, the physician may perform ancillary tests and procedures in order to confirm the presence of salivary gland cancer.

- **Fine Needle Aspiration (FNAB).** In order to accurately diagnose skin cancer, the diagnosis must be confirmed on pathology. This is the diagnostic procedure of choice in all types of thyroid cancer. If the mass can be felt by the clinician, then a small needle can be introduced with an attempt at extracting cells for microscopic assessment. The appearance of abnormal cells will help support the diagnosis of cancer. Sometimes, not enough cells are extracted, and repeat biopsies may need to be performed. This may also be performed with the help of ultrasound or computed tomography (CT) guidance. More recently, genetic testing has been used to help in determining the likelihood of nodules being malignant.

- The extract is usually characterized according to the Bethesda Classification System with an associated risk of malignancy given that result:
  - **Bethesda I**- (1-4% risk) *Non Diagnostic or Unsatisfactory Result.* This refers to insufficient or unsatisfactory sampling, with recommendation for repeat FNAB.
  - **Bethesda II**- (0-3% risk). *Benign* sampling. This indicates that there were no malignant appearing cells.
  - **Bethesda III**- (5-15% risk). *Atypia of Undetermined Significance or Follicular Lesion of Undetermined Significance.* This reveals the presence of atypical or follicular cells, with insufficient information to make a diagnosis of benign or malignant lesion.
  - **Bethesda IV**- (15-30% risk). *Follicular Neoplasm or Suspicion for Follicular Neoplasm.* This indicates that there is follicular cells with an increased likelihood of malignancy.
  - **Bethesda V**- (60-75% risk). *Suspicious for Malignancy.* This indicates an aspirate with a high likelihood of malignancy.
  - **Bethesda VI**- (97-99% risk). *Malignant.* This indicates a diagnosis of cancer.
- **Surgery.** Surgery sometimes is performed in the workup of thyroid cancer. In cases in which a diagnosis cannot be reached based on FNAB, a surgeon may elect to perform a thyroid lobectomy, in which the nodule and the lobe that the nodule is located on is removed and analyzed by a pathologist.
- **Imaging.** Often times a physician may elect to obtain imaging that will help in better understanding the presence of cancer and any other underlying issues
  - **Ultrasound.** Ultrasound imaging is usually the modality of choice in characterizing thyroid nodules. High risk features that indicate a high likelihood of malignancy include calcification or increased vascularity. Ultrasound may also be used in conjunction with FNAB, to assist in localization of a nodule. Ultrasound can also be used to identify lymphatics with disease.
  - **Computed Tomography (CT)**: CT-Scans usually provide a more detailed image of the head and neck region, identifying parts of the tumor that is not readily seen on exam, as well as the presence of regional disease not readily detected (e.g. in the neck). CT-Scans can be obtained with or without contrast. Given the complexity of the region, usually CT scans are obtained with contrast, to help in identify the vascular architecture within the neck. However, this is not always necessary, and CT scans may be obtained without contrast in circumstances that preclude patient receiving contrast (iodine allergies, kidney disease).
  - **Magnetic Resonance Imaging (MRI)**: MRI can also be utilized with or without contrast in order to provide superior visualization of soft

tissue that surrounds the lesion. MRI may be helpful in distinguishing the tumor from surrounding tissue within the head and neck, as well as demonstrate characteristic features that assist in determining its likelihood of being malignant.

- o **18-Fluorodeoxyglucose Positron Emission Tomography (18-FDG PET):** FDG-PET scans may be performed with CT or MRI imaging and are most often used in cases of recurrence..
- **Blood Work.** Blood work may be used in the workup of a thyroid neoplasm.
  - o **Thyroid Function Tests**. These tests may be ordered to determine the level of functioning of the thyroid, and stratify the risk of wheher or not a nodule is likely malignant.

Type of Cancer. Thyroid cancers have varying pathology and behavior. They are often classified according to their level of differentiation, or resemblance to normal thyroid cells.

- **Well Differentiated Thyroid Cancer (WDTC).** These cancers arise from follicular thyroid cells, and closely resemble normal cells in appearance and behavior. These have positive prognosis and outcomes.
  - o Papillary Thyroid Cancer
  - o Follicular Thyroid Cancer
- **Medullary Thyroid Cancer (MTC).** These cancers arise from the parafollicular cells (in contrast to follicular in WDTC), which are responsible for calcium metabolism. These generally are rare, and have a more aggressive course.
- **Anaplastic Thyroid Cancer.** These cancers are the rarest tumor types with the most aggressive behavior, and poorest outcomes.
- **Primary Thyroid Lymphoma.** Lymphomas may arise within the thyroid gland, although relatively rare in incidence.
  - o Non-Hodgkins B-Cell
  - o Mucosal Associated Lymphoid Tissue (MALT)
  - o Hodgkin Lymphoma
  - o Burkitt Cell Lymphoma
  - o T-Cell Lymphoma
- **Metastatic Tumors.** Tumors from other parts of the body may manifest as metastatic disease in skin.

Staging of Salivary Gland Tumors. Once the appropriate diagnosis and work up of skin cancer is complete cancer stage is determined. Currently, the method of staging used is the *American Joint Commission on Cancer (AJCC) Staging Manual* 7th edition.[1] The staging system is broadly referred to the TNM staging system, and is a descriptor of the factors that impact the staging of a cancer.

Staging of Well Differentiated and Medullary Thyroid Cancers[7]

Tumor mass (T). The T staging will characterizes the tumor itself.

- **TX:** Primary tumor cannot be assessed.
- **T0:** No evidence of primary tumor.
- **T1:** The tumor is 2 cm (slightly less than an inch) across or smaller and has not grown out of the thyroid.
- **T1a:** The tumor is 1 cm (less than half an inch) across or smaller and has not grown outside the thyroid.
- **T1b:** The tumor is larger than 1 cm but not larger than 2 cm across and has not grown outside of the thyroid.
- **T2:** The tumor is more than 2 cm but not larger than 4 cm (slightly less than 2 inches) across and has not grown out of the thyroid.
- **T3:** The tumor is larger than 4 cm across, or it has just begun to grow into nearby tissues outside the thyroid.
- **T4a:** Moderately Advanced Local Disease. The tumor is any size and has grown extensively beyond the thyroid gland into nearby tissues of the neck, such as the larynx (voice box), trachea (windpipe), esophagus (tube connecting the throat to the stomach), or the nerve to the larynx. This is also called *moderately advanced disease.*
- **T4b:** Very Advanced Local Disease. The tumor is any size and has grown either back toward the spine or into nearby large blood vessels.

Nodal Status (N): This descriptor is used to describe the presence and number of lymph nodes in the neck.

- **NX:** Regional (nearby) lymph nodes cannot be assessed.
- **N0:** The cancer has not spread to nearby lymph nodes.
- **N1:** The cancer has spread to nearby lymph nodes.
    - **N1a:** The cancer has spread to lymph nodes around the thyroid in the neck (called *pretracheal*, *paratracheal*, and *prelaryngeal* lymph nodes).
    - **N1b:** The cancer has spread to other lymph nodes in the neck (called *cervical*) or to lymph nodes behind the throat (*retropharyngeal*) or in the upper chest (*superior mediastinal*).

Metastatic Disease Status (M): This is used to describe the presence or absence of distant metastatic disease.
- **M0:** No evidence of distant metastatic disease.
- **M1:** Presence of distant metastatic disease.

Final Staging for WDTC. Once a value is assigned to each descriptor of the TNM cancer system, a final stage will be assigned. Age has huge impact on staging, with younger patients (less than 45 doing better).

- Patients Less than 45 years of age

Stage 1 Any T	Any N	M0	
Stage 2 Any T	Any N	M1	

- Patients Older than 45 years of age

Stage 1	T1	N0	M0
Stage 2	T2	N0	M0
Stage 3	T3	N0	M0
	T1-T3	N1a	M0
Stage 4A	T4a	Any N	M0
	T1-T3	N1b	M0
Stage4B	T4b	Any N	M0
Stage 4C	Any T	Any N	M1

Final Staging for Medullary Thyroid Cancer. Once a value is assigned to each descriptor of the TNM cancer system, a final stage will be assigned. Age has no impact.

Stage 1	T1	N0	M0
Stage 2	T2	N0	M0
	T3	N0	M0
Stage 3	T1-T3	N1a	M0
Stage 4A	T4a	Any N	M0
	T1-T3	N1b	M0
Stage 4B	T4b	Any N	M0
Stage 4C	Any T	Any N	M1

Staging of Anaplastic Thyroid Cancer[7]

All anaplastic thyroid cancers are Stage IV. This reflects the poor prognosis and aggressive nature of the disease. Stage IV cancers can be further subdivided.

Stage 4A	T4a	Any N	M0
	T1-T3	N1b	M0
Stage 4B	T4b	Any N	M0
Stage 4C	Any T	Any N	M1

Treatment Plan. Depending on the pathology, site of disease, the clinical staging, and patient factors (co-morbid health conditions, patient preferences) a patient specific treatment plan should be outlined.

- **Surgery.** Surgery is usually the treatment option of choice for all stages of thyroid cancer.

- o **Thyroid Lobectomy.** This type of surgery involves removal of a single lobe of the thyroid containing the lesion. Lobectomies are recommended for early stage well differentiated thyroid cancers, without evidence of aggressive disease. The American Thyroid Association is continuously updating its guidelines and recommendations for lobectomy[8]:
    - Lesions <4cm in size
    - No extension beyond the gland
    - No evidence of extensive involvement of the regional lymphatics
  - o **Total Thyroidectomy.** This type of surgery involves removal of the entire gland and is reserved for aggressive WDTC, anaplastic, and medullary thyroid cancer.
- **Radioactive Iodine.** Radioactive Iodine may be used adjunctively in the treatment of thyroid cancer if there is persistent or recurrent disease.
- **Other Considerations.** Specific attention should be given to the presence or absence of neck disease in the patient.
  - o **Therapeutic Neck Interventions.** If there is any presence of disease within the neck it should be addressed with some type of therapeutic intervention. Positive neck disease is usually treated through surgical resection of the actual positive nodes, and all intervening nodes in the neck.
  - o **Elective Neck Interventions.** In the absence of any clinical evidence of disease, an elective neck intervention may be performed. This means to treat the neck (with radiation or surgery) due to the potential for "occult" or hidden disease that is not clinically apparent. If there is a high likelihood (>15%) of occult disease, an elective neck dissection may be performed.

Prognosis. The prognosis and survival associated thyroid cacner is heavily influenced on the pathology, and the stage of disease.

Well Differentiated Thyroid Cancer

Papillary thyroid cancer[1]

Stage	5-Year Relative Survival Rate
I	Approx. 100%
II	Approx. 100%
III	93%
IV	51%

Follicular thyroid cancer[1]

Stage	5-Year Relative Survival Rate
I	near 100%
II	near 100%
III	71%
IV	50%

Medullary thyroid cancer[1]

Stage	5-Year Relative Survival Rate
I	near 100%
II	98%
III	81%
IV	28%

Anaplastic thyroid cancer[1]

The 5-year relative survival rate for anaplastic (undifferentiated) carcinomas is approximately 7%.

Tracheal Tumors

Overview

The trachea is the portion of the airway that runs through the neck before the bronchial portion within the lungs. Tracheobronchial tumors are exceedingly rare, accounting for 2.6 new cases per million each year and fewer than 1% of all malignancies.[9,10] Due to their close association with the airway detection and management of these tumors is very important. Although treatable in their early stages, these tumors often present during late stages compromising prognostic outcomes.

Causes. Given the rarity of these lesions, there is little definitive knowledge with regards to cause. However, smoking has been considered a risk factor. Other risk factors include history of papillomas within the airway and HPV infection. These tumors may also arise sporadically.

Signs and Symptoms. Signs and symptoms of tracheobronchial tumors may mimic other conditions, such as asthma, making diagnosis difficult and delayed.

- **Asymptomatic.** Tumors in their early stages may be insidious with no symptoms. They may be found as incidental lesions during the workup of other conditions.
- **Breathing Difficulties.** These tumors may present with shortness of breath that may be progressive, or sudden manifesting as severe respiratory distress.
- **Cough.** Patients may present with cough.
- **Coughing Blood.** Tumors may present with blood tinged sputum or frank blood.

Diagnosis and Workup. In addition to routine history and physical examination, the physician may perform ancillary tests and procedures in order to confirm the presence of salivary gland cancer.

- **Diagnostic Bronchoscopy and Biopsy.** Often times when a lesion of the trachea or bronchi is suspected, an operative evaluation will be performed under general anesthesia. This will allow direct visualization of the airway, and provide opportunity for biopsy.
- **Imaging.** Often times a physician may elect to obtain imaging that will help in better understanding the presence of cancer and any other underlying issues
  - **Chest X Ray.** Often times a chest X-ray may be performed in the workup of a tracheobronchial tumor despite being diagnostic in only 50% of tumors.[11]

- o **Computed Tomography (CT)**: Computed Tomography scans are currently the imaging modality of choice for diagnosis of tracheobronchial tumors.[11] It provides details about the airways, regional lymphatics, as well as the lung fields.
- o **Magnetic Resonance Imaging (MRI):** MRI can also be utilized with or without contrast in order to provide superior visualization of soft tissue that surrounds the lesion. MRI may be helpful in distinguishing the tumor from surrounding soft tissue, as well as demonstrate characteristic features that assist in determining its likelihood of being malignant.
- o **18-Fluorodeoxyglucose Positron Emission Tomography (18-FDG PET):** FDG-PET scans may be performed with CT or MRI imaging and are most often used in determining spread of metastatic disease or recurrence.
- **Blood Work**. Blood work may not be necessary, and the decision to obtain blood work is individualized to every patient.
  - o **Liver Function Tests (LFTs):** Can be utilized to determine the presence of concurrent liver disease that may be associated with risk factors for the development of tracheobronchial tumors (alcohol consumption, hepatitis). Furthermore, abnormal values may indicate the presence of metastatic liver disease.
  - o **Complete Blood Count (CBC):** This will identify the presence of any anemia that can sometimes be associated with poor nutrition, or chronic illness.
  - o **Nutritional Blood Work:** If a patient seems nutritionally depleted, particularly in advanced cases, the clinician may elect to obtain laboratory work up to measure nutrition markers in the blood work. This may assist in determining if a patient requires supplemental nutrition.

Type of Cancer. Not all tracheobronchial tumors are malignant, with some being indolent or benign.
- **Benign Lesions**
  - o Papillomas
  - o Tumors arising from the cartilage
  - o Hamartomas
  - o Hemagniomas
  - o Neurilomas
  - o Leiomyomas
  - o Oncoyctoma
  - o Glomus Tumor
- **Malignant Tumors**
  - **Salivary Gland Origin.** The majority of tracheobronchial tumors arise from salivary glands. *(see also Salivary Gland Cancer)*
    - ▪ **Adenoid Cystic Carcinoma** (most common)

- Mucoepidermoid
  - Mucinous cystadenoma
  - Pleomorphic Adenoma
  - **Bronchial Carcinoids.** These tumors arise from a different cell line, more closely related to neurological cells.
  - **Squamous Cell Carcinoma.**
  - **Lymphoma**
    - Mucosal Associated Lymphoid Tissue (MALT)
    - Hodgkin Lymphoma
  - **Metastatic Tumors.** Tumors from other parts of the body may manifest as tracheobronchial tumors.

Staging of Tracheobronchial Tumors. Once the appropriate diagnosis and work up of tracheobronchial tumors is complete cancer stage is determined. Currently, the method of staging used is the *American Joint Commission on Cancer (AJCC) Staging Manual* 7[1] edition[1]. The staging system is broadly referred to the TNM staging system, and is a descriptor of the factors that impact the staging of a cancer.

Tumor mass (T). The T staging will characterizes the tumor itself.

- **TX:** Primary tumor cannot be assessed.
- **T1:** The tumor is 2 cm and confined to the trachea.
- **T2:** The tumor is more than 2 cm and confined to the trachea.
- **T3:** The tumor has extended beyond the trachea but not into any adjacent organs or structures.
- **T4:** The tumor invades adjacent organs and structures.

Nodal Status (N): This descriptor is used to describe the presence and number of lymph nodes in the neck.

- **NX:** Regional (nearby) lymph nodes cannot be assessed.
- **N0:** The cancer has not spread to nearby lymph nodes.
- **N1:** The cancer has spread to nearby lymph nodes.

Metastatic Disease Status (M): This is used to describe the presence or absence of distant metastatic disease.
- **M0:** No evidence of distant metastatic disease.
- **M1:** Presence of distant metastatic disease.

Final Staging for Tracheobronchial Cancer[1]. Once a value is assigned to each descriptor of the TNM cancer system, a final stage will be assigned.

Stage 1	T1	N0	M0
Stage 2	T2	N0	M0

Stage 3	T3	N0	M0
Stage 4	T4	N0	M0
	Any T	N1	M0
	Any T	Any N	M1

Treatment Plan. Depending on the pathology, site of disease, the clinical staging, and patient factors (co-morbid health conditions, patient preferences) a patient specific treatment plan should be outlined.

- **Surgery.** Surgery is usually the treatment option of choice for all stages of tracheobronchial cancers.
  - **Open Surgery.** Open surgery involves resection and reconstruction of all parts of the trachea involved with tumor. This method usually requires the reconstruction of the trachea. This surgery is high risk, with operative mortality of up to 5%.[12]
- **Bronchoscopic Treatments.** In patients unable to tolerate open surgery, with locally advanced disease, or metastatic disease, treatments can be delivered through minimally invasive use of a bronchoscope.
  - **Laser Therapy.** Lasers may allow for tumor debulking, and palliation of any obstructive symptoms from the tumor.
  - **Spray Cyrotherapy.** Application of liquid nitrogen facilitates the disintegration of the tumor.
  - **Photodynamic Therapy.** Utilizes photons from light source to destroy tumor, with minimal impact on surrounding tissues.
  - **Argon Beam Coagulation.** Utilizes argon gas to destroy tumor.
- **Radiation.** Radiation treatment is not routinely used in the definitive treatment of tracheobronchial tumors. Radiation may be an option in poor surgical candidates or in cases of recurrence. Some studies suggest that radiation therapy may be used alone or in combination with surgery in the treatment of adenoid cystic carcinoma.[13]
  - **Brachytherapy.** This is a special type of radiation therapy delivered through a bronchoscope, applying radiation directly to the site of tumor.
- **Chemotherapy.** Chemotherapy may be a treatment option in select cases to slow the growth of tumor, but not as a definitive modality.

Prognosis. The prognosis and survival in patients with tracheobronchial cancer is heavily influenced on the pathology, extent of the disease, and the stage of disease.[10]

Impact of Pathology[10]

Pathology	5-Year Relative Survival Rate

Squamous Cell Carcinoma	12%
Adenoid Cystic	74%
Sarcoma	53%

Impact of Nodal Status[10]

Node Status	5-Year Relative Survival Rate
No Nodal Involvement	53%
Node Positive	10%

Impact of Disease Extent[10]

Disease Extent	5-Year Relative Survival Rate
Localized	47%
Regional	26%
Distant	3%

Radiation Treatment

Radiation therapy utilizes ionizing radiation to target cancer cells within head and neck cancers. The ionizing radiation targets specific cell mechanisms, damaging DNA, and forcing cell death. Although radiation may be harmful to normal surrounding tissues, different modalities and delivery methods attempt to minimize such effects. Radiation can be offered alone or in addition to other interventions, and is dependent on the type of tumor, location, stage, and patient related factors. Dosage of radiation is measured in gray (Gy), and varies on the stage and type of tumor, the setting in which radiation is administered, in addition to location of tumor.

Different Settings of Radiation Therapy

Definitive Radiation (with or without chemotherapy). This type of radiation treatment involves using radiation as the primary mode to treat the tumor. The goals of definitive radiation therapy is complete removal of all tumor with external sources of radiation.

Adjuvant Radiation (with or without chemotherapy). This refers to the use of radiation in combination with surgery. The goal of adjuvant radiation is to treat any remaining disease after surgical removal (e.g in circumstances with positive margins).

Neoadjuvant Radiation (with or without chemotherapy). Radiation given prior to surgery is referred to as neoadjuvant radiation. This is not routinely performed in the treatment of oropharyngeal cancers and is used in academic centers as part of larger studies.

Methods of Delivery

Conventional External Beam Radiation Therapy (EBRT). This type of therapy involves the use or X-rays or gamma rays delivered from an external source to a pre-mapped area involving the tumor. Patients are placed in a specifically calibrated machine in which the regions of treatment are simulated/planned. A treatment plan is generated by the radiation oncologist, and delivered over the course of several weeks to achieve the desired affects. Intensity Modulated Radiation Therapy (IMRT) involves the use of EBRT in conjunction with CT and MRI scans that allo for 3-Dimensional mapping of the region to be treated. This minimizes effects to surrounding normal and vital structures, maximizing delivery to the tumor.

Stereotactic Radiation. This is a specialized form of EBRT also known as Radiosurgery in which high concentrations of radiation is delivered to focused regions of tumor.

Brachytherapy. Brachytherapy involves the use of radiation seeds or catheters implanted at the site surrounding the tumor. These implants allow for the slow delivery of radiation to a well-defined tumor area over a prolonged period of time. This type of radiotherapy is limited in its application to only well defined tumors that are slow-growing. The implantation and removal of the implants may require a surgical procedure.

Intraoperative Radiation Therapy. This type of radiation therapy may be offered at some institutions, and is reserved for patients that have received and failed previous radiation therapy, or cancers that involve highly critical structures (brain, skull base, carotid arteries). This type of therapy is delivered in the operating room after the removal of tumor, and focuses the radiation to a specific field. This will minimize effects to surrounding tissue that have been previously treated that would not tolerate any further radiation exposure. Such treatments may take 30 minutes, followed by completion of the surgical procedure.

Radioactive Iodine. This is a form of radiosurgery specifically used in the treatment of thyroid cancer. Thyroid cells are the only cells in the body capable of trapping and taking up iodine. Taking advantage of this, radiation can be attached to Iodine molecules and administered to a patient, such that all thyroid tissue, including those harboring cancer will take in the radioactive element resulting in cell death. This type of therapy is used after complete surgical removal of the thyroid gland with evidence of recurrence or persistent disease.

Effects of Radiotherapy

Radiation has far reaching effects on the normal tissues within the head and neck. Although radiation oncologists attempt to minimize these effects by limiting exposure to normal tissue, these side effects still develop. These side effects may be acute or late.

Acute Side Effects. These side effects tend to occur throughout the course of treatment, or immediately following completion of treatment.
- **Nausea and Vomiting**
- **Dryness of the nose, mouth, and throat**
- **Sores in the nose, mouth, and throat**
- **Dryness and irritation of skin**

Late Side effects. These side effects occur well after completion of treatment (months to years) and are related to the fibrosis and scarring of involved tissues.
- **Skin Changes.** Skin becomes less elastic and more firm, giving a "woody" quality. Radiation also impacts sweat glands reducing sweat formation.
- **Epilation.** Hair loss.

- **Dryness.** Radiation has impactful changes on the salivary and lacrimal (eye) glands of the head and neck causing xerostomia (dry mouth), and xeropthalmia (dry eye).
- **Cancer.** Radiation may pose a risk factor for development of subsequent malignancies due to their ionizing effects on DNA. Specifically, patients have an increased risk of developing thyroid cancer.
- **Swallowing Problems.** Radiation may cause stenosis of the esophagus, or dryness of the lining of the digestive tract, reducing swallowing abilities.
- **Hypothyroidism.** Radiation may reduce the ability of the normal thyroid to function normally.

Chemotherapy and Other Anti-Tumor Medications

Chemotherapy involves the use of medications target cancer cells at the site of tumor as well as in distant tissues. These medications target cells that are replicating tumor cells that replicate at fast attempting to arrest their growth. However, these medications inadvertently also target normal cells that replicate fast such as hair cells, or cells within the skin of lining of the stomach, resulting in side effects. Chemotherapy can be administered through intravenous infusion (IV), intramuscular (IM) injections, orally, or through skin (for skin cancers).

Settings in which Chemotherapy is Administered

The use of systemic medications is used adjunctively with either surgery or radiation, and is used to target disease distant from the local site. It is not used as a primary treatment modality as it does not facilitate eradication at the primary site. Chemotherapy is often used in circumstances of advanced disease (Stage III or IV), or when certain risk factors for distant disease are present. Such risk factors include lymph nodes with disease that have extended out of their capsule (not contained), positive surgical margins, or involvement of nerves.

Induction Chemotherapy. This refers to chemotherapy performed prior to surgery or radiation. This may be used to see the biological response of the tumor to chemotherapy, as well as "shrink" tumors to a manageable size that can be better removed with surgery or radiation.

Adjuvant Chemotherapy. This refers to chemotherapy given after definitive treatment with another modality was performed (either surgery or radiation).

Concurrent Chemotherapy. This refers to the decision to administer chemotherapy and radiation concurrently after surgery. This may be the case in situations of predictors of aggressive disease on pathology.

Palliative Chemotherapy. This involves the use of chemotherapy for palliation of symptoms in cases that cannot be cured. This type of treatment may slow cancer progression, attenuating the tumors impact on quality of life functions.

Chemotherapeutic Agents

The most commonly used chemotherapeutic agents are cisplatin, carboplatin, 5-Fluorouracil, hyroxyurea, paclitaxel, docetaxel, and epirubicin. Depending on the type of cancer, stage, and recommendations of a medical oncologist, these agents may be used alone or in combination with one another.

Side Effects

The majority of side effects are related to the impact of the chemotherapeutic agent on normal tissues.

- **Nausea and Vomiting**
- **Hearing Loss**
- **Swallowing difficulties**
- **Ulcers in the nose, mouth, and throat**
- **Kidney Failure**
- **Rash**
- **Hair loss**
- **Infertility**
- **Sexual Dysfunction**
- **Fatigue**
- **Weight Loss**
- **Predisposition to life threatening infections**
- **Diarrhea**

Functional Implications Following Head & Neck Cancer: An Overview

Unfortunately, head & neck cancer frequently affects many of functions we use daily for normal survival such as breathing, eating and talking. It is not uncommon for one or more of these abilities to be affected both during and after cancer treatment. In many cases, alternate means of talking, eating and even breathing may be required. Comprehensive and aggressive rehabilitation by knowledgeable and experienced specialists is required to allow for as normal as function as possible following treatment.

The following information is provided as a general guide to some of the functional deficits and associated treatments that are common in the head & neck cancer population. The information is divided into sections addressing the various functional issues that may arise both during and after cancer treatment. Following each section are some commonly asked questions you may find helpful. Every patient experience, however is unique and should be evaluated and treated on an individual basis. An open conversation with your speech-language pathologist (SLP) will allow for realistic expectations regarding functional outcomes.

Surgical Recovery: Optimizing Outcomes

If surgery is required for your cancer treatment, there will often be functional deficits affecting swallowing, voice and speech. Adequate healing must occur before an evaluation and any rehabilitation measures can be conducted. It is important to follow the post-operative care instructions provided by your doctor and SLP to ensure the best recovery possible.

In addition to the structural affects of surgery itself, scarring from surgery, **several months later**, may result in a decline in function, -especially regarding speech and swallowing. Your SLP will likely provide you with exercises and stretches to use following a period of healing. Following the exercise guidelines for several *months* post-operatively will ensure the least impact from surgical scarring.

As with any wound, surgical wounds in the mouth/throat will heal best if kept clean and free from irritating factors. For this reason, you may not be able to eat by mouth for a period of time following surgery as food/liquid intake will irritate and contaminate the wound. In some cases, you may require a swallowing test to determine what is safest for you to swallow before you resume eating by mouth. Once cleared to resume eating, you may be limited to softer foods or even liquids for a period of time. For optimal recovery and safety, it is very important that any dietary restrictions be closely followed.

Additionally, it is always best to adhere to a low-acid diet. Acidic food and drink can interfere with wound healing, may potentially increase wound pain and prolong the overall return to function. In general, adhering to a low-acid diet for six weeks post-operatively is advised.

Low-Acid Diet

☐ Avoid spicy foods, sauces and condiments

☐ Avoid vinegar and anything pickled

☐ Avoid fruits and fruit juices (melons and bananas are ok)

☐ Avoid tomatoes and anything made with tomatoes (red sauces, ketchup, etc)

☐ Avoid alcohol

☐ Avoid coffee

☐ Avoid all sodas and carbonated beverages

Radiation Care

In many cases, radiation (and possibly chemotherapy) will be recommended as part of your cancer treatment. Radiation treatment affects everyone differently although side-effects of radiation treatment fall into both **acute** *(short-term)* and **latent** *(delayed)* categories. While the acute effects usually resolve in the weeks following completion of treatment, the latent effects may evolve several months or even years following radiation. Research has shown that **what you do during radiation greatly affects how you swallow after treatment.** For this reason, your SLP will conduct "radiation counseling" prior to initiation of your radiation treatment. This will detail exercises, dietary guidelines as well as nutrition and hydration goals to allow for the best possible outcome following radiation.

Swallowing During Radiation Treatment

In general, it is VERY IMPORTANT to continue to eat by mouth during radiation. Although many patients have a g-tube placed prior to heading into radiation, this tube should only be used to supplement what you are eating/drinking by mouth and ONLY as needed.

Keep Swallowing!

The muscles of the throat are similar to muscles in the other parts of the body. When these muscles are not used as much as they are used to, they begin to weaken. This is part of normal muscle physiology. Now consider the effects of radiation, most notably, *fibrosis,* which can be thought of like scar tissue in that it is tougher and less flexible than healthy muscle fibers. This fibrosis takes hold between the muscle fibers, and can limit how much they are able to move. For this reason, it is very important to keep the muscles moving during treatment.

Exercise Your Swallow

In most cases, patients can have difficulty eating as they typically would during radiation treatment. Additionally, the acute effects of radiation may be interfering with how well you are able to swallow. For this reason, swallowing exercises are very important to maintain swallowing function *even after radiation is completed.* Your SLP will give you a list of exercises to perform at least twice daily during radiation and the first weeks following treatment.

Jaw Stretches

Unfortunately, radiation can have a significant impact on jaw opening. In some cases, surgery prior to radiation can also limited how wide you are able to open your mouth. For these reasons, it is very important to conduct regular stretching exercises for your jaw. As a general rule, you should be able to insert three fingers vertically between your teeth. If you are unable to do this, contact your doctor/SLP.

What to Eat

Your SLP may give you specific instructions on what you should eat, although the general guideline is to **eat as normally as possible!** The body knows how much effort to exert when swallowing. For example, it takes more "muscle" to swallow a piece of meatloaf, than it does to swallow a sip of milk. Although the pain of radiation may cause many patients to consider limiting themselves to liquids, the bulkier the food you swallow, the more you are working the throat muscles.

The radiation effect to the esophagus is also important here. At rest, the esophagus is like a slender, flexible tube. As bulky foods move through, it stretches to expand around it as needed. Consider how a snake body expands around its prey when eating. Same thing! The upper portion of the esophagus is within the radiation field when the neck is being targeted. For this reason, it is important to swallow more bulky foods to ensure the regular "stretching" of this part of the esophagus. In this way, you are helping to discourage the fibrosis from taking a strong hold on the flexible muscular fibers of the esophagus.

Ouch! When it Hurts to Swallow

Odynophagia is a term used to describe painful swallowing. Most patients experience odynophagia to some degree at some point during radiation as well as during the recovery period.

Odynophagia is important as it begins to impact not only what you feel like eating, but how well you are able to swallow. In general, odynophagia is the biggest reason most people feel they need to step down their diet, or even consider using the feeding tube. Your SLP staff can work with you to help find food choices that can minimize your pain when eating. Odynophagia can also be helped significantly by using special anesthetizing mouthwashes before meals. Your radiation oncologist can help you with this more.

Odynophagia also, however, has an impact on how effective the swallow is. In general, when it hurts to swallow, there is a tendency to have a weaker swallow. For this reason, many patients feel they cannot swallow as well. This usually, however, has more to do with the pain they experience. By managing the pain, it may allow for better swallow function. For this reason, if you are experiencing odynophagia, let your oncologist or SLP know so they can work with you to optimize what/how you eat.

Your SLP will determine what you should be swallowing. Try to follow this advice as closely as possible. In general, most patients will alter their diets during radiation. Working closely with your SLP can ensure you are eating foods to help maintain your swallow as much as possible. Switching to the Low Acid Diet can also be very helpful.

"I Don't Have an Appetite"

A loss of appetite is extremely common during cancer treatment as well as recovery. There are several reasons patients lose their appetite during this time. It is important to understand that eating and appetite may no longer have a connection during your treatment/recovery period. It is important for you to eat well and sufficiently, whether by mouth or through a feeding tube, regardless of how hungry you may/may not be.

Nausea can be controlled with medications although it is important to notify your doctors or SLP staff if nausea is a significant issue. There is also medication to assist with improving appetite, but in most cases, patients are encouraged to eat regardless of appetite.

Think of eating like homework. Although you may not want to do it, you need to.

Nothing Tastes Right

Dysguesia is a term used to describe an altered sense of taste. In many cases, patients, can experience a loss of taste, where it becomes difficult to detect any flavor in the food. In other cases, many patients can report food tastes bad. Although some of the dysguesia may be a result of surgical changes, there may also be some neurologic impact of radiation to the nerves coming from the taste buds.

Although we have historically enjoyed food for its flavors, it's important to continue eating even when food has lost its attraction. Not only is proper nutrition important for normal body function, it is especially important in helping to keep up your strength. Without proper nutrition, the body is not able to recover/heal as well following radiation as well.

Although it is nearly impossible to avoid some of the long-term affects of radiation, doing your part to keep everything working can help to ensure you remain as functional as possible after your treatment is completed and into the future.

Xerostomia

Xerostomia is a term used to describe dry mouth and it is a very common side effect of radiation treatment. In many cases, the salivary glands are impacted by radiation treatment and this causes both a decrease in salivary production as well as a change to the viscosity of the saliva, most often becoming thicker and less moisturizing.

Swallowing is designed to be a lubricated event, with saliva providing the lubrication required to allow food to pass efficiently through the mouth and throat. Without this natural lubrication, dry foods will always have more difficult passage through the throat.

Additionally, while there is less saliva for lubrication, the saliva is produced is thicker and stickier. In essence, these altered secretions can actually serve to hinder the swallow instead of helping to lubricate. Think of the throat as being coated in tacky glue. In some cases, this can be the effect of the altered secretion production.

Although this may improve somewhat following recovery from radiation, there is typically a permanent change to the moisture level of the mouth and/or throat, depending on the focus of radiation. Although there is no way to reverse these effects, there are some medications that may help improve salivary production. Your doctors can discuss these options with you.

Swallowing with Xerostomia

Although the saliva production cannot be replaced, it is important to ensure a safe and effective swallow that lubrication is still present. The following tips can help improve your swallow outcome when you are experiencing dry mouth

- Adhere to a SOFT MOIST diet, avoiding dry textures
- Use extra sauces and gravies to help moisturize/lubricate the food you are eating
- Avoid bread, this sticks to the drier surfaces of the mouth/throat
- Chew thoroughly so there are no "chunks" as these are the most likely to not pass as well through the throat.
- Alternate solids with liquids while eating. Using liquid swallows to wash the food down can help move the food through a dry throat.
- Swallow several times per bite. It's harder to swallow through a dry throat so the more you swallow, the more likely you are to effective move the food into the esophagus.

As always, if you are noticing increased difficulty swallowing, you are coughing or choking when you eat or feel like you are not able to eat enough by mouth, you should always contact your SLP for further evaluation. In many cases they can find ways to help you and ensure the safest and most effective way to eat.

Compensating for Xerostomia

Findings ways to compensate for the xerostomia is very important. While there are certainly comfort concerns, the mouth and throat are lined with tissues that are designed to stay moist. Taking sips of water, if cleared by your SLP, can assist in maintaining adequate moisture in the mouth and throat. Some patients find hard candies are helpful in this regard as well, although typically, you should avoid any containing peppermint, cinnamon, or ascorbic acid (lemon/sour flavors) as these may cause increased irritation to the mouth and throat.

There are also commercial products designed to help with xerostomia. The Biotene line of products is specifically designed for patients with xerostomia.

Many patients have also found Oasis oral spray to be helpful in improving dry mouth comfort. Your pharmacist can assist you in locating these products.

Improving the humidification, especially at night can also help with the extreme dryness many patients report after waking in the morning. As most adults breath through their mouth when sleeping, the mouth and throat can become extremely dry and parched. Using a humidifier by the bed will help to provide moisture to the air you breath in while sleeping.

Nutrition During Radiation Treatment

Many patients experience some weight loss during the course of their cancer treatment. This can be the result of many factors including loss of appetite, difficulty swallowing, pain, loss of taste and generally not feeling well. Your doctors and SLP staff will closely monitor your weight during this time to ensure you do not become critically malnourished.

In general, your calorie needs are the same or even greater than they were before your cancer diagnosis. Although you may not be as active, during treatment, your body continues to need the same energy (calories) to deal with the effects of radiation as well as to properly heal/recover. Proper nutrition is key for immune system function as well as in allowing for adequate and timely healing/recovery.

Eating by Mouth

What to Eat

Your SLP will determine what you are capable of eating/drinking safely and they strive to prescribe the most normal texture diet possible. The intake of solid foods is extremely important, when possible. It ensures the highest level of muscle activity when you swallow and, in doing so, helps to preserve your muscle strength and function, both during and after your treatment. It is important to eat the solid foods your SLP has indicated are safe for you.

The body knows how much effort to exert when swallowing. For example, it takes more "muscle" to swallow a piece of meatloaf, than it does to swallow a sip of milk. Although the pain of radiation may cause many patients to consider limiting themselves to liquids, the bulkier the food you swallow, the more you are working the throat muscles.

The radiation effect to the esophagus is also important to consider here. At rest, the esophagus is like a slender, flexible tube. As bulky foods move through, it stretches to expand around it as needed. Consider how a snake body expands around its prey when eating. Same thing! The upper portion of the esophagus is within the radiation field when the neck is being targeted. For this reason, it is important to swallow more bulky foods to ensure the regular "stretching" of this part of the esophagus. In this way, you are helping to discourage the fibrosis/scarring from taking a strong hold on the flexible fibers of the esophagus

How Much Should I Eat?

Your SLP may give you specific instructions on what you should eat, although the general guideline is to **not lose weight**. Nutritional supplements may be advised by your doctor or dietitian, if you are not eating enough to sustain your weight.

Many patients ask how much they should eat. The answer? AS MUCH AS YOU CAN! The texture of the foods may change, as your SLP may counsel you. The foods you eat may also change to ensure the safest and strongest swallow possible. But a general guideline is to eat enough to maintain your weight.

In some cases a combination of tube feeding and eating by mouth is required. When you are unable to eat enough by mouth, you may be counseled to use your feeding tube as well. It is very common for patients to eat by mouth as well as use their feeding tube. Eating by mouth is always the preferred method, if it's safe to swallow. But getting enough nutrition and hydration is the ultimate goal. Sometimes, it becomes necessary to use the feeding tube to boost your overall nutrition and hydration. Always discuss this with your SLP so they are able to best advise you. They will work with you to preserve your swallow ability as much as possible, while also ensuring you are receiving proper nutrition/hydration.

How Often?

Most patients find their eating habits are altered significantly during radiation treatment. Eating smaller portions more frequently through the day may provide you with the best overall plan for eating. How often you eat is of little concern as long as you are taking in enough nutrition to maintain your weight and stay properly hydrated.

Water/Hydration

During radiation, we recommend to our patients that they have a **gallon** of water daily. Although this seems like a lot, your body has a much higher need for water during your treatment.

It's always better to drink it (use that throat!) if you have been cleared to drink water. But if drinking this much is too difficult, or you are not able to drink by mouth, then use the feeding tube to take in the water. How you get the water in you is less important than being sure you get the full gallon into your body.

Consider this: Compare a pile of wet firewood with a pile of dry firewood. Now try burning each pile. The wet wood doesn't burn so easy. Now think of this in terms of your tissues. The better hydrated you are, your body acts more like the pile of wet wood, more resistant to the burning effects of radiation. If you don't have enough water in your system, your body responds more like the pile of dry wood, often experiencing more severe radiation effects.

You will notice secretions becoming thicker during radiation. This effect becomes worse if the body is not well hydrated. Drinking water, therefore, can help keep this effect better managed. In addition, the dry mouth that can result from these thicker secretions can be greatly relieved by taking small sips of water. Be sure your SLP has cleared you for drinking water if you are using a feeding tube.

Frequently Asked Questions

I know it's important to keep swallowing during radiation but is there a certain amount I should be sure to eat each day?

You should eat as much as possible by mouth. There is no predetermined amount of oral intake and patients are encouraged to take as much by mouth as possible. If you are able to drink a can of tube feeding, it's always better to drink it than to put it through the tube.

When will I feel the effects of radiation?

In general, the acute effects are radiation begin to become prominent during the third week of treatment. For this reason, monitored care by you SLP will general happen during week three or four, after some of the more notable effects are being experienced. In this way, your symptoms are monitored and care plans may be altered as such to ensure the best possible functional outcome.

How long will it take to recover from radiation?

Just as the effects of radiation are observed to come along gradually, the recovery is also more gradual. Generally, speaking, three weeks after completion of radiation treatment, many of the acute effects are greatly diminished. There are, however, more long term effects of radiation that can be lifelong in duration. These may begin to be more notable following recovery from the acute phase of your treatment. Your doctor or SLP staff can discuss this with your more thoroughly.

Why is my mouth so dry?

Xerostomia is the term used to describe the dry mouth experience may patients notice during as well as after radiation. This happens when the salivary glands are impacted by the effects of radiation. Both the amount of output from these glands as well as the consistency of the saliva is changes. There is typically less saliva generated and it can be more viscous, or thicker than before. Although this may improve somewhat following recovery from radiation, there is typically a permanent change to the moisture level of the mouth and/or throat, depending on the focus of radiation.

When will my sense of taste return?

Dysguesia is a term used to describe an altered sense of taste. In many cases, patients, can experience a loss of taste, where it becomes difficult to detect any flavor in the food. In other cases, many patients can report food tastes bad. Although some of the dysguesia may be a result of surgical changes, there may also be some neurologic impact of radiation to the nerves coming from the taste buds.

How directly the taste buds are exposed to radiation determines to some extent, how quickly your sense of taste will return. If the tongue is a direct target, it may take several months for your sense of taste to return. Despite this, the return of function is gradual so you may begin to notice some sense of taste after a few weeks. This should continue to improve over time.

Why do I have so much mucous?

In response to radiation injury, *mucositis* can develop, which is an inflammation of the mucous membranes, resulting in excessive mucous production. This is also very thick in nature and therefore can be more difficult to manage. Using a humidifier as much as possible can be helpful as drier air can cause the mucous to become thicker and stickier. Ice chips and sips of water can help break up the mucous although you should check with your SLP before doing this is you are not eating by mouth.

Feeding Tubes

A feeding tube is a means by which you are able to receive nutritional support (food/liquid) into the stomach or intestinal tract while bypassing the mouth and throat. For head & neck cancer patients, feeding tubes are commonly used for a variety of reasons. Some of these are detailed below, although if you have questions or concerns regarding the use of a feeding tube, your doctor or SLP should be able to answer your specific questions.

Why Feeding Tubes are Used

There are many reasons why a feeding tube may be used. Although many patients may be reluctant to have a feeding tube, understanding the benefits of the tube, as well as the risks associated with *not* using a feeding tube, may help with this decision.

Post-operative Recovery

Any more extensive surgery impacting the mouth or throat will require the use of feeding tube for at least the post-operative recovery period. It is important the surgical wounds are not exposed to contamination by food/liquid during the recovery process, which may interfere with wound healing and even lead to infection.

Ongoing Cancer Treatment

Many head & neck cancer patients require chemotherapy and/or radiation during the course of their treatment. Adequate nutrition is key in promoting good endurance as well as healing. During the course of treatment, it may not be possible to take in sufficient nutrition/hydration by mouth. In these cases, the feeding tube can be helpful to adequately nourish and hydrate the patient.

Dysphagia

This is a term used to describe a problem with the patient's ability to safely and effectively eat/drink by mouth. Dysphagia can occur for a variety of reasons in the head & neck cancer population. In most cases, rehabilitative methods to restore the ability to swallow are implemented as quickly as possible. However, depending on the severity of the dysphagia, a feeding tube may be required to ensure nutritional needs are safely met during rehabilitation.

Your doctor and SLP will determine when it is ok for you to return to eating by mouth

Types of Feeding Tubes

There are three main types of feeding tubes commonly used. The classification of the tubes refers to the route or pathway of the tube itself. There can be multiple variations of each type of tube and your doctors will determine which is best for you.

Nasogastric Tubes (NG Tube)

These are tubes generally used for more short-term purposes. These tubes are placed through the nostril, pass through the throat, through the full length of the esophagus and end in the stomach or small intestine. These tubes do not require surgical placement, although their placement is typically checked with an x-ray before used for feeding to ensure adequate situation in the stomach/intestine.

Because these tubes are placed through the nose, they are generally not indicated for long-term use (>30 days) as this placement can become uncomfortable and cumbersome.

Gastrostomy Tubes (G-Tube)

These tubes are typically placed when a more long-term need for tube feeding is anticipated. These tubes are surgically placed into the stomach and held in place by an inflatable cuff. G-tubes can be concealed easily beneath clothing and are therefore much less conspicuous than an NG tube. A G-tube can be indicated for use over several weeks to several years, although generally should be replaced every six months. Although the initial placement is surgically done, replacement of the tubes is easily done in an office setting and is virtually painless.

Jejunostomy Tubes (J-Tube)

These tubes are typically used for the same reasons a g-tube would be used, although this is surgically placed further down the digestive tract, into the *jejunum*, which is a portion of the small intestine near the stomach. The j-tube is typically only used when a g-tube cannot be placed, although the reasons for this vary greatly. A more common reason a j-tube is used is to reduce the potential for *gastroesophageal* reflux, which occurs when stomach contents leave the stomach and pass into the esophagus, the opposite direction food should travel through the digestive tract. If this problem is severe, your doctor may opt for a j-tube placement. Other reasons include abdominal surgery, which may have altered the gastrointestinal tract. Your doctor will determine which tube is most appropriate for you, depending on your individual needs. Like the g-tube, the j-tube can be used for several weeks to several years, although will require periodic replacement.

Enteral Feeding Methods

Feeding Tube Food

When you first start the tube feeding process, a specific canned formula will usually be prescribed to you by your doctor or registered dietitian. These formulas are designed to best meet your individual nutritional needs. It is important to feed the amount prescribed (number of cans per day) as well as the additional water that may be indicated. This is a convenient method of feeding as it requires little preparation. These formulas, however, may be difficult to tolerate and can result in nausea, vomiting and diarrhea. Should this occur, your dietician can try various formulas to improve tolerance.

Head & neck cancer doctors are also advocates of using regular food, -anything you'd typically eat, that is nutritious. Nearly any food can be processed in a blender using fluid (milk, chicken broth, canned formula). This should be blended until smooth and thin enough to be passed through the tube. In this way, it's possible for the patient to "eat" the same meal their family is eating. In the event canned formulas are not well tolerated, this may present a very good option.

Feeding Tube Pumps

A feeding tube pump is a machine, similar in nature to an IV pump, whereby the formula is delivered to the stomach at a set amount over the course of several hours. A pump may be used during the initiation of the tube feeding process, allowing for a gradual adjustment to this new way of "eating." In some cases, prolonged use of a pump is used when larger volumes of food cannot be delivered to the stomach.

Gravity Bags

A gravity bag is similar to a feeding tube pump in that it allows for the formula to be delivered slowly over time. Bags do not require a separate pump to function and for many patients, provide a convenient alternative to the pump.

Bolus Feeding

Most patient's typically transition from the pump method to bolus feeding. This term is used to explain when larger volumes of food are delivered through the feeding tube in a relatively short period of time, similar to how we eat meals. A typical bolus feeding may consist of two cans of formula, or a normal sized meal that has been properly processed.

Bolus feeding more closely resembles normal nutritional delivery. Our bodies are used to having full meals delivered to the stomach. For this reason, as well as the cumbersome nature of being connected to a feeding pump, patients are encouraged to transition to the bolus feeding method.

Gastrostomy Tube Troubleshooting

Pain At The Tube Site

Pain at the tube site may be caused by a variety of reasons. The most common of these is tissue irritation by stomach acid that has seeped from the stomach into the tube tract. This can often be helped by medication but it is important your doctor assess the exact cause of the irritation and pain before treating. If you notice increased pain, irritation, bleeding or pus at the tube site, it is important to be evaluated by your physician.

Broken End Tips

There are no replacement parts for gastrostomy tubes. If an end cap is missing, a foam earplug can very effectively be substitutes to seal the tube ends. These can be purchased at any pharmacy very inexpensively. These should only be used as temporary plugs until you are able to see your physician and have the g-tube replaced. They will, however, spare the frustration of a leaking g-tube until replacement is possible.

Clogged or Slow Passage

It is very common for food material residue to build up along the wall of the gastrostomy tube. If this build-up becomes significant, it can dramatically slow the passage of material through the tube and potentially cause it to clog. Flushing the tube regularly with water can help. Coca-Cola has also been found to be highly effective in dissolving this residue but is more effective on smaller amounts of residue. Waiting until the residue becomes significant may mean it is very difficult, if not impossible to effectively clear the tube.

In the event a clog occurs and it is impossible to pass any material through the tube, it is important you seek medical attention quickly, especially if you have not been cleared to take anything by mouth and the g-tube is the only way of taking medications and nutrition.

Frequently Asked Questions

What is a Feeding Tube?

A feeding tube is a tube through which you are able to receive nutritional support (food/liquid) into the stomach or intestinal tract while bypassing the mouth and throat. Any extensive surgery involving the mouth or throat will likely require the use of a feeding tube for at least a short time. During the post-operative recovery/healing process, it is important the surgical wounds are not exposed to food and liquid, which would interfere with healing and potentially lead to infection. If the swallowing mechanism is no functioning properly (there are a variety of reasons), a feeding tube may also be advised.

Can I still eat by mouth if I have a feeding tube?

Yes! Having a feeding tube does not mean you cannot eat by mouth, although you should always follow the advice of your doctor and/or SLP staff regarding how much you should be using your tube. Your SLP staff will determine what foods and how much of them you can eat safely.

If I can eat by mouth, why do I need a feeding tube?

There are many reasons a feeding tube is placed even when the patient is able to eat by mouth. In some cases, the feeding tube is placed in anticipation of needing it during the course of your cancer treatment. In many instances, the feeding tube can help supplement the patient's overall nutrition if what is eaten by mouth may not be enough to adequately nourish the patient.

Why am I being changed from an NG tube to a G-tube?

In most cases, an NG (nasogastric) tube is placed when the need for tube feeding is anticipated to be short-term. There are however, instances where the need for tube feeding appears as if will be more long-term in nature (>30 days). In these instances, placement of a g-tube is advised as this is more comfortable, can be left in place as long as necessary and is generally easier to maintain and less conspicuous. Once the g-tube is placed, the NG tube can be easily removed.

Can I shower/bathe with a G-tube or J-tube?

In most cases, you can shower 48 hours after the tube placement. Bathing is usually ok after 10 days although you must be cleared by your surgeon before bathing.

When can my g-tube be removed?

When considering g-tube removal, your doctors/SLP will first determine there will be no further cancer treatment and/or surgery planned that may require use of the feeding tube. Even if further treatment may be several weeks away, your g-tube will not be removed, although you may not need to use it except for daily flushing.

Once your SLP has determined that you are able to safely eat by mouth *enough to maintain proper nutrition/hydration,* you will be instructed on proper weaning from the feeding tube. You will be monitored to ensure you are maintaining your weight and hydration. After this is demonstrated, your feeding tube can be removed.

Swallowing and Dysphagia

Normal Swallowing

Swallowing is a complex and coordinated activity that requires various muscle groups and other structures, including the larynx, to function in a swift and coordinated manner. When this doesn't happen properly, it can result in food or liquid falling into the trachea, known as "aspiration." This is what happens when a person chokes.

To briefly describe a normal swallow, of course it begins in the mouth. This is referred to as the *oral phase* of swallowing. During this phase, you chew any solid food and your tongue works in coordination with your lips and cheeks to organize the material in your mouth and move it, all together, to the back of the mouth, or the *oropharynx* (where the mouth joins the throat).

Once this happens, the *pharyngeal phase* of swallowing occurs. During this phase is when much of the work of swallowing is accomplished.

The tongue base pushes backward and downward, making contact with the superior pharyngeal constrictors. These are the highest muscles in the throat. This begins the downward movement of the food material toward the esophagus. As this happens, material fills the *vallecula.* This is a "pocket" in your throat created on one side by the tongue base and by the *epiglottis* on the other side.

As the tongue base pushes downward, the pharyngeal constrictors begin to contract, like a purse string, from the top of your throat downward in a wavelike manner. At the same time, muscles connected to the larynx and hyoid bone, pull the larynx upward and slightly forward. The vocal cords also close during this to protect the windpipe from food going in.

The closing of the vocal cords also plays a very important role in the swallow process. By closing, they prevent any air from leaving the lungs during the swallow. This *subglottic pressure* is important for driving a strong swallow.

As the larynx moves upward, two other very important things happen. The epiglottis flips backward or *retroflexes* over the opening to the larynx, like a lid covering the larynx and trachea during the swallow. While this helps to protect the airway from food material entering, it also allows for the tongue base to now clear the food out of the vallecula. As the epiglottis flips backward, the vallecular pocket turns into a smooth slide, deflecting the food material past the protected larynx and downward toward the esophagus.

Another important action happens when the larynx moves upward and forward during the swallow. This action also pulls open the *cricopharyngeus*, or "upper esophageal sphincter" which remains closed except during swallowing, burping or vomiting. This is a small muscle at the top of the esophagus that opens to allow food and liquid to pass, then closes to prevent reflux or regurgitation back into the throat. At rest, the cricopharyngeus is closed.

The entire time, the pharyngeal constrictors work in conjunction with these other actions, squeezing in a purse string manner from top to bottom. The middle pharyngeal constrictors are active when moving the food past the larynx. The inferior pharyngeal constrictors help to squeeze the food material past the cricopharyngeus and into the esophagus.

Once into the esophagus, the *Esophageal Phase* of swallowing begins. The esophagus is a tube like muscular structure that squeezes from the top downward in a wavelike manner called *peristalsis*. This action is what moves the food into your stomach.

Dysphagia

Dysphagia is the term used to describe a disorder involving any/all phases of swallowing. Depending on the extent and severity of the dysphagia, a patient may be required to change what they eat, how they eat, or use an alternate means of nutritional delivery entirely (i.e., feeding tube).

Your SLP will perform comprehensive evaluations to determine if you are experiencing dysphagia. They will also determine the reasons for this and how best to manage the dysphagia. This may include therapy, diet changes and/or ways of eating differently.

When assessing dysphagia, your SLP considers two primary concerns:

1. **Swallow Safety:** When the swallow is not normal, it is possible for food, liquid and even the body's own secretions that are typically swallowed to fall into the airway and lungs. This is known as *aspiration*. Patients may or may not realize this is happening! The lungs and pulmonary airways are sterile environments in the body. Any aspirated material introduces bacteria into the lungs. This can potentially lead to infection and even death. It's also possible to choke, blocking the airway entirely and leading to asphyxiation. Aspiration is a primary concern in dysphagia. Your SLP will evaluate the swallow function and provide instructions for eating to allow for the safest intake of food. For this reason, it is very important to closely follow those instructions.

2. **Swallow Efficiency:** For most people, a meal can be eaten quickly, over the course of several minutes. In the presence of dysphagia, however, the swallow efficiency may be compromised, meaning it will take a longer than standard period of time to consume food/liquid. If there is very poor swallow efficiency, the patient may be physically incapable of taking in enough nutrition by mouth to meet their individual needs. This is also a very important consideration when assessing dysphagia and your SLP will provide eating instructions with this in mind. For example, although it may be *safe* for you to eat a regular diet (i.e., no elevated aspiration risk), if it takes a very long time to chew more solid foods, you may be instructed to stick to a SOFT diet to allow for better efficiency.

Because dysphagia may place you at an increased risk for aspiration as well as nutritional compromise, it is very important to follow the guidelines for eating set forth by your SLP .

Common Symptoms of Dysphagia

The symptoms listed here are the most commonly reported although any perceived difficulty eating/swallowing should be reported to your doctor or SLP for further evaluation.
- coughing/choking during meals
- drooling
- Longer than standard meal times
- Sensation of food/liquid remaining in the throat following the swallow
- Regurgitating solids after attempting to swallow
- Food/liquid coming through the nose
- Painful swallowing

Any one of these symptoms is sufficient to warrant a swallow evaluation and many patients may experience several of these symptoms simultaneously. Regardless of how many symptoms may be present, it is important to have an objective swallow evaluation conducted to determine the presence of dysphagia, the apparent causes, possible treatment options and appropriate feeding guidelines to ensure safe and efficient nutritional intake.

Evaluating Dysphagia

Fiberoptic Endoscopic Examination of Swallowing (FEES)
During this examination, a flexible nasopharyngeal fiberscope, as used by the physicians in the office, is passed into the throat. The throat is then thoroughly examined and may be tested for sensitivity as well as reflexes (cough and swallow).

Dyed food samples are then used to test the swallow ability across a variety of different textures. In doing this, the SLP is able to determine if there is normal swallow function or if there is a dysphagia. If dysphagia is present, the SLP will assess why the swallow is not normal, what can be safely eaten by mouth, if tube feeding is warranted and what necessary treatment is needed to improve the swallow.

Following the examination, you will be thoroughly counseled regarding findings, eating recommendations and necessary interventions to improve the swallow function.

Modified Barium Swallow

This examination requires use of fluoroscopy, a type of x-ray, and for this reason, cannot be done in an office setting.

For this examination, various textures of barium are used to test the swallow ability across a variety of different textures. In doing this, the SLP is able to determine if there is normal swallow function or if there is a dysphagia. If dysphagia is present, the SLP will assess why the swallow is not normal, what can be safely eaten by mouth, if tube feeding is warranted and what necessary treatment is needed to improve the swallow.

Following the examination, you will be thoroughly counseled regarding findings, eating recommendations and necessary interventions to improve the swallow function.

Clinical Swallow Examination

This is a non-instrumental examination conducted by the SLP. During this examination, various food textures and liquids may be testing with clinical observations made. In this practice, a clinical examination is not frequently performed as instrumental findings can be more valid, especially in the presence of surgical changes. Often this is done when there is very little suspicion of dysphagia.

Management of Dysphagia

Once a dysphagia has been diagnosed, proper management is critical to the patient's health as well as to maximize their overall function in regard to swallowing.

In this practice, there are three main ways we manage dysphagia: dietary changes, intake modifications, and therapy. Typically, most patients are prescribed a combination of these three although each management plan is unique in addressing the specific needs of every individual patient/circumstances. Your SLP will detail the management plan using the following components:

Dietary Guidelines

Your SLP will thoroughly explain, as well as provide written information, regarding the dietary guidelines you are to follow. This addresses the types of foods you eat, how much to eat at one time and how often you should eat. If you have questions regarding how certain foods may/may not be appropriate to eat, you should always ask your SLP before including in your diet. Although these provide a basic overview, any specific questions you have should always be addressed to the staff. The Dietary Guidelines at the end of this section provide specifics regarding each dietary level.

Intake Modifications

Your SLP will thoroughly explain specific instructions for *how you eat/drink.* Using intake modifications often allows patients to eat a higher level diet (more regular diet) than they may be safely able to without the modifications. For example, a patient may be able to eat a Puree diet well, although has more difficulty when foods are not pureed. However, your SLP has determined that through the use of multiple swallows and alternating liquids, more solid foods can be just as safely eaten.

It is very important to use the intake modifications you are prescribed. In most cases, these modifications, along with the dietary guidelines, are what will allow you to eat in the safest and most efficient manner. Failure to comply with the modifications and dietary guidelines as prescribed can be dangerous to your health. Your intake modifications will be explained and a list of these will also be provided to you to take home. Only use the modifications prescribed to YOU! Attempting to use alternate modifications may be extremely unsafe!!!

Dysphagia Therapy

Your SLP will determine if you are an appropriate candidate for rehabilitation of your swallowing disorder. In most cases, therapy will be recommended to begin immediately. There are instances, however, when initiation may be delayed. Some common reasons for delaying therapy include:

- Additional surgery is pending
- Additional wound healing is required
- Other more urgent health concerns are present
- Extreme physical debilitation
- Concurrent radiation treatment

In addition to office based therapy, there are also therapy programs designed to be home programs (conducted independently by the patient), as well as combination programs which have both office-based and home components. The combination programs are the most commonly prescribed as these allow for continued work outside the office, while the office based-therapy provides the main work and structural framework for the treatment.

The premise for therapeutic intervention is to provide effective rehabilitation which will allow for the safest, most efficient swallowing at the highest level possible. There are frequently limitations to how much progress can be made in therapy and realistic expectations will be communicated following your initial dysphagia evaluation.

Depending on the progress you demonstrate, your course of therapy may be continued, extended or discontinued. In general, as long as improvement is being demonstrated, your therapy will continue. Once improvements are no longer made, when you have reached a *therapeutic plateau*, then consideration to discharge will be given. In this practice, however, a small course of therapy may be continued after maximum gains are made to ensure the long-term effectiveness of your therapy.

It is very important to understand that the continuation of therapy vs discharge from therapy is based on *improvement of function* and NOT what you are eating/not eating. Resuming a normal diet is NOT the goal of therapy. Rather, getting a patient to swallow as *best as possible* is always the goal. This may or may not include returning to a regular diet. Your SLP is very good in explaining realistic expectations of therapy. If you have any questions in this regard, do not hesitate to ask.

Strength and Range of Motion Exercises

In many cases, a dysphagia is caused by a muscular issue, whereby certain muscles have weakened or have been surgically removed, either partially or completely. In these instances, it is critical to strengthen the muscles as much as possible. We typically provide exercises to be done at home, three times a day. These comprise either a home based program, the home component for a combination program, or even the office based program itself. Your SLP, however, will introduce you to these exercises and ensure you are able to complete these properly before instructing you to conduct these at home. Your SLP will also determine your course of therapy in this regard.

Neuromuscular Electrical Stimulation

In order to utilize this form of treatment, the SLP must be FDA certified to administer this therapy modality. This is an aggressive, office-based therapy during which electrical stimulation is applied to various targeted muscles in the throat, causing contraction of the muscles. This can be very effective although your SLP can direct you more regarding realistic expectations from this treatment modality.

While this treatment can be very effective, it can also be painful, -although it varies widely from patient to patient in this regard. Your SLP will work with you to ensure your comfort as much as possible. There are specific instructions to follow that will ensure optimal comfort.

Therapeutic Progress

Your progress/improvement will be monitored at regular intervals throughout your therapy with an objective/instrumental swallow evaluation. This serves several purposes:

- To determine if therapy techniques are "working"
- To identify therapy needs/goals for the next course of treatment
- To advance your diet as much as possible

If therapeutic progress is made, then swallow function should also be improving. How quickly this is happening and in what areas you are improving can vary greatly from person to person. However, once swallow ability has improved to allow for changes in what/how you are eating, your SLP will change your diet and intake modifications accordingly. It is important to follow these guidelines since what you eat/how you eat can also serve to augment your therapy, improving your progress even more! This is especially important if you have been cleared for *therapeutic feeding,* as this serves as a transitional phase from g-tube reliance to eating by mouth again.

Returning to Eating Again

Often times, patients are very anxious to eat by mouth following a prolonged period where they had to rely on feeding tube nutrition. This can quickly be replaced with feeling of anxiety as the realization is made that swallowing is now very different.

Fear of choking is a normal and natural response. It's important to understand, however, that your SLP has had years of extensive training and education in this regard. They are your resource for learning about your swallowing problem, determining what you can/can't safely eat, and developing a plan for rehabilitation.

Realistic goals will be discussed although they may be adjusted as therapy continues. In some cases, the patient progresses beyond what was expected and other times, there may be slower progress appreciated.

As you continue along the rehabilitative process, your SLP will provide you with all the information you need to support your rehabilitative goals, including how to wean from your feeding tube as your swallow function improves.

Many patients are anxious to have their feeding tube removed as soon as possible, however, only your doctor/SLP can determine if and when this is appropriate for you. Once g-tube removal appears to be an appropriate consideration, you will be asked to wean from using it and/or stop using it for feeding entirely. *Continue to flush your tube daily until it is removed, even if you are not using it.*

Your weight and intake will be monitored once you stop using the feeding tube. If this remains stable, consideration of removal may be warranted. Your doctor/SLP can discuss option in this regard.

Dietary Guidelines

SOFT DIET

What is a soft diet?

Being on a soft diet means that the foods you eat will need to be soft enough to easily cut with a fork. In general, if it makes a noise when you bit into it, you likely shouldn't be eating it! Foods made with ground meats as well as pastas and casseroles are examples of some common soft food items. Tougher meats such as steak and chicken should be avoided unless they are very tender. In some cases, it may be better to avoid these meats completely but your Speech Pathologist will discuss this with you.

Helpful Hints

It will always be easier to eat foods on a soft diet when they are well moistened. You may like to use extra sauces, gravies and syrups to moisten your foods. If you need to use thickened liquids, be sure to follow the guidelines for how thick these items should be.

Try to avoid anything crunchy. Often, soft casseroles will have a crunchy topping that may be difficult to manage for someone on a soft diet. Other soft foods such as French toast or pancakes may develop hard crusts. These should be softened by soaking in a liquid such as syrup or removed entirely before eating.

Foods to AVOID

Some foods will always be difficult to swallow safely if you are on a soft diet. The following items should be avoided:

- Jello
- Nuts and Seeds
- Crisp Bacon
- Raw vegetables
- Crisp fruits
- Dried fruits
- Corn, popcorn
- Chips and other crunchy foods
- Dry cereals

If there are certain foods you know you have a difficult time swallowing, you should always avoid them, even if you do not see those items listed above.

PUREED DIET

What is a pureed diet?
Being on a pureed diet means that the foods you eat will need to be blenderized until they are smooth and resemble pudding or mashed potatoes. You are usually able to have your favorite foods as long as they have been pureed first.

How do I make pureed foods?
All foods should first be cooked as usual. Place food items in the blender and press the "puree" button. Continue blending until the food is smooth and resembles pudding. THERE SHOULD BE NO CHUNKS. Often, juice or broth may need to be added to the food items when blenderizing to make sure they are smooth and pudding-like. Certain foods, such as cooked fruits and vegetables, will turn runny when pureed. In this case, potato flakes or another thickening agent should be used until mixture is pudding-thick. If you also need to use thickened liquids, use the same thickener to make sure that all foods are at least as thick as your liquids are required to be.

Foods to Avoid
Some foods will always be difficult to swallow safely if you are on a soft diet. The following items should be avoided:

- Jello
- Nuts and Seeds
- Rice
- Bacon
- Fruits and vegetables with skins
- Dried fruits
- Corn, popcorn
- Chips and other crunchy foods
- Dry cereals

If there are certain foods you know you have a difficult time swallowing, you should always avoid them, even if you do not see those items listed above.

MOIST DIET

What is a moist diet?
Being on a moist diet means that the foods you eat will need to be soft enough to easily cut with a fork. In addition, these foods should also have a great deal of moisture in them or added to them before you attempt to swallow. Foods made with

sauces, gravies, as well as pastas and casseroles are examples of some common moist food items. Tougher meats such as steak and chicken should be avoided unless they are very tender. In some cases, it may be better to avoid these meats completely but your Speech Pathologist will discuss this with you.

Helpful Hints

If you have been prescribed this diet, it will always be easier to eat foods when they are well moistened. You may like to use extra sauces, gravies and syrups to moisten your foods. This can be especially helpful to request in restaurants. If you need to use thickened liquids, be sure to follow the guidelines for how thick these items should be.

Try to avoid anything crunchy. Often, soft casseroles will have a crunchy topping that may be difficult to manage for someone on a moist diet. Other soft foods such as French toast or pancakes may develop hard crusts. These should be softened by soaking in a liquid such as syrup or removed entirely before eating.

Using sips of liquid can also be very helpful to someone following a moist diet. Taking frequent sips of liquid can assist with providing the extra needed moisture/lubrication to the swallow. It is very easy, however, to become full quickly when you take in lots of fluid simultaneously. If this happens, you should be sure the liquid you are drinking has good nutritional value, such as Boost or Ensure.

Foods to AVOID

Some foods will always be difficult to swallow safely if you are on a moist diet. The following items should be avoided:

- Jell-O
- Nuts and Seeds
- Crisp Bacon
- Bread
- Tortillas
- Raw vegetables
- Crisp fruits
- Dried fruits
- Corn, popcorn
- Chips and other crunchy foods
- Dry cereals

If there are certain foods you know you have a difficult time swallowing, you should always avoid them, even if you do not see those items listed above.

Thickening Liquids at Home

If your Speech Pathologist has determined that you are at risk for fluids going "down the wrong way" and entering your lungs, you may be required to utilize thickened liquids.

Thickening Agents

There are various commercial thickening agents that are readily available at most pharmacies. The most common of these are powders that can be added to nearly any liquid. "Thick-It" and "Thicken-Up" are two such commonly found products. There are also other thickeners as well as ready-to-drink products available online. Your SLP can assist you with this if you like.

A less expensive way to thicken liquids is by using potato flakes or baby cereal. When added to liquids, these will also thicken well. These may take a bit more blending to achieve a smooth texture and the taste may be different than when using a commercially designed product.

Levels of Thickened Liquid

There are three distinct levels of thickened liquids:

Nectar Thick (Level I)
Honey Thick (Level II)
Pudding Thick (Level III)

Of course, if you are thickening liquids yourself, there can be variations somewhere between the level (i.e., Thicker than nectar but still thinner than honey). As long as the liquid is *at least as thick* as what you are prescribed, it's ok. You must thicken to level you are prescribed or more. Follow the directions on the thickener label to thicken to the appropriate consistency when using a commercial product. Trial-and-error will work best when using potato flakes/baby cereal as these respond differently to different liquids.

What Should Be Thickened

All thin liquids need to be thickened before you eat or drink them. Here is a list of liquids that must be thickened:

- Water
- Juices
- Milk
- Egg Nog
- Soda Pop
- Soups
- Coffee and Tea (hot or iced)
- Hot Chocolate

- Thin Gravies and Sauces
- Nutritional supplements (Ensure, Boost, etc.)

Things to Avoid

Some food items are difficult to swallow safely when you must use thickened liquids. Other food items produce juices when chewed and should also be avoided. Here is a list of items to avoid while you are required to thicken your liquids:

- Jell-O
- Popsicles (melts to a liquid)
- Milk Shakes (usually ok for Nectar Level diets)
- Ice Cream and Sherbet (usually ok for Nectar Level diets)
- Ice and Ice Chips
- Slushes and Smoothies
- Canned Fruits (full of juice)
- Vinegar based salad dressings (too thin)
- Juicy Fresh Fruit
- Tomatoes (too juicy)

THERAPEUTIC FEEDING

The benefit of therapeutic feeding allows you to experience limited oral intake while exercising the muscles of swallowing. This allows for a degree of oral gratification from an NPO status (nothing by mouth) , as well as serve to provide some gradual strengthening and rehabilitation of the weakened musculature. This will augment your therapy with the potential for speeding your overall recovery. For this reason, it's very important to follow this protocol.

Your SLP will advise you if you are allowed cold food/liquid. It's always advised to avoid cold food/liquid for the first 3 months following surgery where there has been flap reconstruction. You will be cleared by your doctor or SLP for cold foods.

What/How to Eat

Only eat TWO OUNCES of pudding per session. These sessions should be conducted four times per day. If you purchase prepackaged pudding, each session you will eat ½ container. You will go through two containers per day. The flavor of these does not matter but it must be SMOOTH pudding (not rice, bread or tapioca puddings).

Follow these instructions for eating:

1. Swallow ½ teaspoon of pudding per bite
2. Swallow each bite three times
3. Follow with 1 teaspoon of liquid, by spoon

4. Cough
5. Repeat

Any difficulty with this should be reported to your SLP so they can make appropriate changes and ensure the safety of your swallowing.

Remember, this is your treat AND your homework!!

Trismus

When a person is unable to open their mouth a normal amount, they are diagnosed with *trismus*. Although there are several potential causes of trismus, the most common cause in this practice is the result of surgery and/or radiation changes affecting the temporomandibular mandibular joint, the joint connecting the mandible (lower jaw bone) to the skull.

In this case, inflammation of the joint structures and/or radiation fibrosis can make the jaw opening very limited. There are other cases where muscle spasm may cause the joint to be very resistant to opening as well.

While trismus can be very uncomfortable for a patient, it can also result in serious function problems, depending on severity. Without the ability to open the mouth fully, patients may have a very difficult time maintaining proper oral hygiene, especially when the mouth opening is too small to fit a toothbrush.

Eating can also become difficult if the mouth opening is too small to fit a food-laden fork or spoon. Chewing can become difficult without sufficient space between the teeth. Eating whole fruits, sandwiches and the like can also be difficult when the mouth is unable to open large enough to bite into these foods.

Speech production can also be greatly impacted since the tongue has less room to move when articulating, or making different sounds. Consider trying to speak with your mouth shut. This is very typical of what a trismus patient experiences when there is minimal to no mouth opening.

Trismus Management

Prevention

Prevention of trismus is a primary focus. Certain radiation targets, such as the tongue, tonsil and oropharynx can often result in trismus. As such, identifying patients at a high risk for developing trismus allows us to prescribe an exercise regimen designed to minimize the effects of radiation to the temporomandibular joint.

By executing these exercises provided by the SLP department on a consistent and regular basis, you help to prevent some of the effects of radiation that may result in more severe trismus. Although it is often impossible to avoid developing some degree of trismus, by executing the prescribed exercises on a regular and consistent basis, you help to prevent temporomandibular joint implication as much as possible.

Therapy

Despite following prescribed preventative measures, it is often impossible to avoid developing at least some degree of trismus following radiation treatment for tongue, mandible, tonsil and oropharynx cancers. If trismus is diagnosed and considered to impact your *functional* abilities (i.e., ability to eat, speak, etc), therapy may be indicated to improve your jaw opening as much as possible.

Passive stretching exercises are most commonly used to assist with improving mouth opening. Your SLP will guide you through a program best designed to meet your needs, which may include the use of splinting devices, Therabite, a passive range of motion device, or the Dynasplint which incorporates counterbalance measures to assist with jaw opening. Your SLP can discuss the available options in this regard as well as identify the best device for your individual needs.

Therabite

The most commonly utilized device for treating trismus is the Therabite Jaw Rehabilitation System. It is important to note that regular exercise with this system is required to achieve and maintain any gains in mouth opening.

Dynasplint

This system can be effective in improving jaw opening although is less commonly used as this device is rented and requires custom fitting by the manufacturer. Its utilization of counterbalance principles can be very effective in improving mouth opening.

Botox

In some cases, trismus can be caused by, or made worse, by muscle spasms within the temporomandibular joint. In this case, the use of Botox may be helpful to assist with the management of your trismus.

Although Botox can be quite effective, it will not help trismus that is the result of radiation fibrosis or other causes. It is *only* effective in treating muscle spasms that may be interfering with mouth opening. Your doctor/SLP staff will determine if this treatment is appropriate for you.

If spasm is suspected to be interfering with mouth opening, electromyography (EMG) will first be used to assess the degree of muscle activity (spasm) within the joint to help determine if this course of treatment is appropriate for you.

It is important to understand that the effects of Botox are not permanent. Ideally, Botox should last 3-4 months although the effective time is different from patient to patient and dependent on several variables. Repeated injection can be performed as the effects of Botox begin to wear off to ensure your trismus is well managed.

Surgery

In some cases, surgery can be performed to assist with mouth opening, although following surgery, passive range of motion exercises are typically required to maintain the gains accomplished by the surgery. Without regular exercise of this manner, the trismus may potentially return to the same severity as was noticed pre-operatively. Your doctor/SLP will determine if surgical intervention is appropriate for you.

Speech Difficulty

Speech production can be impacted by cancer affecting either the *structure* or the *nerves* that serve the structures important in producing speech. For this reason, even a thyroid or salivary gland cancer can result in communication problems.

Affected structures

Although the tongue is the most common structure known to affect speech production, speech *intelligibility* (how understandable your speech is to others) can be impacted by changes to the oral cavity in general, -even if the tongue is intact. In addition to the tongue, speech production requires the use of lips, teeth, cheeks, hard and soft palates as well as the upper portions of the throat for speaking. If any of these structures are altered by surgery or other treatment, it may affect your speech production.

Therapy can often help improve your speech production, however, once articulatory organs (the structures used to speak with) are altered, "normal" function may not be possible. The goal of therapy is to achieve the highest level of intelligibility for every patient. This may not mean your speech sounds perfect, but rather, as understandable as possible. Your SLP can discuss realistic expectations in this regard.

Consider this example: if you had part of your thumb removed, you'd likely experience some difficulty using your hand as you did before. But with therapy and practice, you could learn to use your hand in a very effective way, and do most of what you could do before; but it would be *different* from when you had all fingers intact. The same is true of the mouth and throat. The remaining structures may still be able to accomplish many of the same functions, but it will need to be in a different manner. This is why therapy is important as it can help you regain your abilities following cancer treatment.

Regardless of your treatment plan, the best therapy for speech is TALKING. As with other things, practice allows for improvement. By writing or not talking much because you don't like how your speech sounds will only hinder your recovery and therapeutic progress.

Treatment/Therapy

In many cases, the most effective therapy may not involve intensive/frequent visits with your SLP or therapist. In some cases the most effective therapy requires consistent and regular practice, -far more frequent than what could be accomplished through office visits. In fact, many times the majority of the work accomplished through therapy is done by you *in the comfort of your own home*. Your personal treatment plan may require practice 7 or more times per day for the best outcome! For this reason, it is best if you are able to do your exercises independently at home once you are instructed by your therapist during office visits. In many cases, office visits may be spaced apart to allow you to practice/strengthen sufficiently before the next level of therapy can be achieved.

Every patient presents with unique abilities and therapeutic needs. A thorough evaluation is required to assess function and determine the most appropriate treatment plan.

Each treatment plan is tailored to suit the individual based on:
1) What the problems are (speech, voice, swallowing, etc)
2) What the limitations are (surgical changes, nerve impairment, etc.)
3) What remains intact
4) How readily a patient can learn the exercises and techniques necessary

Common therapy techniques include exercises and/or stretches. You may be asked to repeat words and/or phrases several times. Whatever is prescribed, it is very important you follow the treatment plan as closely as possible to ensure the best outcome.

Your overall speech ability will be dependent on many factors. Having realistic expectations is important and your SLP should have an honest conversation with you in this regard at the outset of therapy. The best possible outcome is *only* possible with complete collaboration between the patient and the SLP.

KEEP IN MIND: Every patient is unique. Even two patients with the *same* surgery and cancer treatment for the *same* tumor in the *same* structure may have *very different* functional abilities and difficulties. It is important to only follow the treatment plan prescribed for you. If you have questions regarding your treatment, you should always address them with your SLP.

Voice Care

The voice we have, and *how* we make a voice, is typically not anything we pay much attention to, *unless* it begins to fail us. Understanding how a voice is made as well as how to take care of your voice is key in ensuring the best possible quality and reliability of your voice, especially following cancer treatment.

Even if the vocal cords are not directly impacted by cancer, radiation treatment can have a lasting impact on the voice. Changes in your voice may be normal or an indication of a problem. Understanding proper voice care is an important component in your cancer care.

Phonation: Not Just the Vocal Cords

Phonation refers to the process by which we make a voice. While most people believe a voice is produced by the vocal cords, the vocal cords are actually only part of the process. Producing a voice is actually a highly coordinated action that also involves the lungs, the muscles of respiration (breathing) as well as the muscles of the larynx (voice box). When we make a voice, all of these work together to produce the sound we hear.

The quality of the voice produced, therefore, is dependent on several different variables. If one of these components is not working properly, the voice produced may not sound "normal." When you notice a change in your vocal quality, this is a signal there has been a change somewhere in the system.

How a Voice is Produced

The vocal cords, of course are very important in producing a voice. They are positioned at the top of the *trachea*, or windpipe, and have the ability to open and close.

When we breathe, the vocal cords are open, but they come together in order to make a voice or *phonate.* The vocal cords coming together, however, will not result in a voice. In fact, the vocal cords *do not vibrate independently*. In order to produce a voice, the vocal cords must come together, while *simultaneously*, air from the lungs is exhaled through them in a sufficient manner. The flow of air through the closed vocal cords causes vibrations...the sound we hear as a voice!

Consider how leaves rustle in the wind. Vocal cords vibrate like leaves in the wind. Without airflow or "wind," the vocal cords are still, and no sound will be produced. In this sense, you can understand then, how we exhale the air is just as important as the vocal cords in terms of producing a voice.

The quality of your voice is determined by both the health/function of the vocal cords (or vocal *folds)*, as well as the airflow through them. If any of these factors are implicated by either cancer or treatment, you may likely experience a change in your vocal quality.

It is the *quality* of the vocal cord vibration that determines the *clarity* of the voice. Vibratory quality is affected by many factors including the tone/stiffness of the vocal folds as well as the symmetry of the vocal folds (they should be identical in terms of size, shape and tone).

Another determining factor in this regard is the airflow dynamic through the closed vocal folds. Without enough exhaled air, there will be poor vocal fold vibration and a poor voice as a result. If there is an obstruction or other factor limiting airflow in the region of the upper trachea, this may result in altered vibration of the vocal folds and a change in voice will be noted.

Cancer directly affecting the larynx will most likely result in voice changes; but because of the complexity of how a normal voice is made, even cancers and treatment not affecting the larynx or vocal folds can result in voice changes. Some of the more common implications of head & neck cancer treatment that may affect the voice are described here.

Dysphonia: When Hoarseness Should Be Addressed

Dysphonia is a general term referring to an abnormal voice. Dysphonia usually happens to everyone at some point, and typically resolves without intervention. One common example of this is a laryngitis that may occur with a virus. As the virus resolves, the voice usually returns to normal on its own.

There are times, however, when dysphonia does not improve. In those cases, it is good to see your doctor. In general, a dysphonia may not be an indication of a serious health issue, but it may not improve, or may even become worse, without proper diagnosis and care.

Although changes in the voice are common and rarely worrisome, there are indications when voice changes should prompt you to see your doctor:
- Dysphonia that lasts more than 2-3 weeks without any sign of improvement
- Dysphonia that begins without a reason (no illness, etc)
- Voice changes that get worse over time
- Loss of pitch range
- Loss of volume
- Loss of voice control
- Sudden voice changes

Any patient with a history of head and neck cancer should contact their doctor immediately if they notice any of the following voice symptoms:

- Pain when voicing
- Changes in your voice
- Dysphonia and simultaneous ear pain
- Dysphonia and difficulty breathing
- Dysphonia and interference with breathing
- Dysphonia and coughing up blood (even small amounts)

Although there may be nothing worrisome present, it is always best to have your doctor evaluate your symptoms.

Evaluating Voice Changes

Your medical history, as well as your typical voice habits, onset and progression of dysphonia, etc. are all very important information in determining a diagnosis and management plan for your dysphonia. Following a general otolaryngology examination, usually including fiberoptic endoscopic examination of the larynx, further stroboscopic evaluation of your dysphonia will typically be performed.

Stroboscopy

Stroboscopic examination is key to establishing the *etiology,* or cause, of the voice disorder, which then allows for proper management. Although your doctor may have used a flexible fiberscope (through the nose) to examine your larynx, stroboscopy offers a higher level of examination when there is concern regarding the voice and/or the general health of the larynx.

For this examination, a microphone resembling the end of a stethoscope will be secured around your neck. A rigid endoscope is then placed into the mouth and passed to the back of the throat. A lens at the end of the scope allows for a magnified examination of the larynx, beyond what is possible with the flexible fiberscopes used more commonly.

Once the scope is in position to view the larynx, you will be asked to make a voice. During this time, a strobe light will allow for visualization of the actual vocal cord vibrations. It is the use of the strobe light that makes this examination different from other endoscopic examinations. The vocal cords vibrate at a very high speed, making it impossible to observe the vibrations with the naked eye.

Consider watching a hummingbird's wings while it is hovering. Although it is clear the wings are moving, they are doing so too quickly to see with any clarity. The same is true of the vocal cords during phonation. Being able to see these vibrations through the use of stroboscopy allows for a comprehensive examination of your phonatory pattern.

The larynx is capable of producing a voice in many different ways. For example, you can speak softly, shout, sing and laugh. For this reason, when assessing voice issues, it is important to also see what the larynx is capable of doing. Identifying areas that are not considered to be "normal" can be very important in determining a proper diagnosis and management plan. Measuring change and/or improvement in these areas is also helpful in determining the success of treatment. In some cases, a baseline evaluation will be conducted prior to your cancer treatment to assess for any change that may follow.

As part of your voice evaluation, you may be asked to perform certain tasks during which your SLP will be taking measurements and making observations. These will include your typical speaking frequency (pitch), how much you can vary the pitch of your voice, how loud you can be, how long you can sustain a voice, etc. All of this information can be very helpful in assessing your dysphonia, determining proper treatment and then tracking change/improvement based upon those initial measurements.

Types of Voice Disorders

Cancer treatment can impact voice production on several differently levels and can have many different causes. The type of voice difficulty you have will largely determine the appropriate treatment and for this reason, it is extremely important to understand the reason(s) for the voice disorder. In some cases, there may be various options for treatment and your doctor and/or SLP will educate you thoroughly in this regard.

There are two main types of voice disorders, although it is not uncommon to have a combination of the two. In some cases, an organic disorder can result in the development of a functional disorder. For this reason, the best management of your voice disorder may be a combination of treatments.

Organic Disorders

An organic disorder refers to a problem with the mechanisms of phonation and are classified into two categories:

Structural:
A structural disorder refers to a problem with the voice mechanism itself. In this case, there may be fluid in the vocal cords, polyps/cysts interfering with closure and vibration, etc.

Neurogenic:
A neurogenic voice disorder refers to a disruption in the nerves controlling the larynx. Common examples of this include complete or partial vocal cord

paralysis. There can also be spasms in the laryngeal musculature that interfere with the ability to produce a voice.

Functional Disorders

A functional voice disorder refers to a problem with the *manner* in which a voice is produced and can be affected on many different levels. Voicing, or *how we produce a voice,* does not require conscious thought or effort. This is because a signal is sent from the brain that automatically results in the coordinated pattern/event we call voicing. For various reasons, however, this pattern can become altered, resulting in behaviors that are interfering with the production of a clear voice.

In some cases, a functional disorder may arise as a result of an organic disorder. For example, if a vocal cord cyst is interfering with the closure of the vocal cords, there may (unconsciously) be more force or effort to close the vocal cords in light of the obstruction. This extra muscle effort can result in a functional disorder, especially if it is continued over an extended period of time.

Functional voice disorders may also have an inconsistency to them, becoming better or worse at different times. It is even possible to have a very normal voice at times, while at others, a significant dysphonia may be present.

Although there may be a degree of variability noted in organic voice disorders, this dysphonia tends to be more consistent.

Management of Voice Issues

After a comprehensive evaluation, a management plan will be discussed by your SLP. The plan is designed to provide the most effective voice rehabilitation on an individual basis. Of course, the cause of the voice problem largely determines the management. Your doctor and SLP are in close collaboration regarding the best plan for improving your voice and will thoroughly explain the details of your management plan.

Essentially, management can fall under three categories: therapy, medical management and/or surgery. Often times, a combination of approaches is used to achieve the best outcome for your voice.

Voice Therapy

For most functional voice disorders, as well as many organic disorders, voice therapy is indicated to improve phonatory production. The SLP is highly skilled in therapeutic techniques to evoke and maintain the best vocal quality possible.

Although voice therapy can be very effective in improving functional voice disorders, the key to success is patient consistency and participation. Because this type of therapy is aiming to change behavior patterns, consistent practice is required to "reset" those patterns.

The SLP will work with you during your office-based therapy sessions, teaching techniques aimed at improving your phonatory pattern. The office sessions, however, are only a portion of your therapy program. Following each session, you will be provided with a "Home Program." This represents, in essence, your homework, or home practice that must be conducted. Effectively and consistently conducting your Home Program exercise is key to the success of your voice therapy.

How long you are enrolled in therapy depends on the nature and severity of your voice disorder, as well as how quickly your voice responds to therapy. In some cases, patients may require only one or two session while others may be enrolled in therapy for several months.

Your SLP can discuss plans for therapy, including an *estimation* of how long you will participate in therapy. It is important to remember that this is merely an estimation based on typical anticipated responses to treatment. Foreseeable changes in the length of your therapy course will be discussed with you as the need arises.

Medical Management

In some cases, a voice disorder may be caused or exacerbated (made worse), by a medical issue. Some common examples of this are sinus drainage and acid reflux, both of which may result in vocal cord inflammation. Smoking can also cause changes to the vocal cords that will result in a dysphonia. In such cases, therapy alone will not improve the quality of the voice as the overall health of the larynx will need to improve.

Changes in behaviors (such as quitting smoking) may be advised in such cases, although it is not uncommon for medications to also be prescribed. For example, allergy medicines may be prescribed if nasal drainage from allergies is suspected to be contributing to the dysphonia. Similarly, anti-reflux medications may also be prescribed if laryngopharyngeal reflux is thought to be contributing to your dysphonia.

Your doctor/SLP will discuss any appropriate medical management as it may contribute to the rehabilitation of your voice. Following their instructions in this regard will be very important in the overall rehabilitation of your voice.

Surgery

Depending on the nature of the voice disorder, your doctor/SLP may recommend surgery. Although there are many cases where surgery is not appropriate or advised (i.e., can make the voice disorder worse), there are other cases where surgical intervention will be required in order to improve your vocal quality.

Surgery is never indicated for functional voice disorders without an organic component. Not all organic voice disorders, however, require surgical intervention.

In some cases, a combined approach using both therapy as well as surgery is necessary to restore the best vocal function.

Because surgery is an invasive procedure that may have the potential for scarring the vocal cords, it is only considered when other alternatives will not be effective in restoring the voice. Surgery will only be advised when it is believed to provide the best outcome potential, either alone or when combined with other management options.

Common Voice Disorders Following Cancer Treatment:

Most voice disorders arising from cancer treatment are organic in nature although a comprehensive evaluation by an SLP is required to adequately diagnose this. In some case, the voice issue may be temporary in nature and a full recovery of normal vocal quality can be expected. In other instances, the voice changes may be more permanent in nature and your SLP will determine an appropriate means of optimizing you vocal quality.

Vocal Fold Paralysis vs. Fixation

If a vocal fold is paralyzed, either partially or completely, it is not able to move as it needs to in order to close/vibrate against the other vocal fold to produce a voice. In this case a very soft, breathy voice may be noted. Patients may say they "run out of breath" when talking and can no longer generate a loud voice. In some case, a higher pitch voice is noted.

Paralysis/Paresis

The nerves that serve the larynx can sometimes be affected by tumors/surgeries that have nothing to do with the larynx or vocal folds. This is because the nerve *pathway* may be near an affected site. Every possible precaution is taken to ensure the nerve is both identified as well as protected from the surgery as much as possible. Despite this effort, simply the act of retracting the nerve to keep it outside the surgical field can result in impairment. In some cases, a complete vocal fold paralysis may exist. In other cases, there is movement but it is not full function. In most cases, nerve function returns in a few days or weeks. There are some instances, however, when nerve impairment may be more long-standing or even permanent.

Fixation

Radiation treatment can sometimes impact how well the larynx is able to function. Depending on the tumor site, the radiation may directly affect the larynx. These patients are more prone to laryngeal damage from radiation which may result in impaired movement of the vocal folds.

Many structural components of the larynx are made of cartilage, which is the same tissue that forms the structure of the nose and ear. Unfortunately, cartilage can sometimes be damaged by radiation, resulting in "distortion," warping or even fusion in some cases.

Within the larynx, the *cricoarytenoid joint* allows the vocal folds to move as they should. They remain open during respiration, and close during voicing, coughing and swallowing. If the cricoarytenoid joint is damaged as a result of radiation treatment, the vocal fold will not be able to move as it should. Radiation can effect one or both joints, meaning one or both vocal folds may not move as expected. In most cases, radiation effects to the cricoarytenoid joint are not reversible, but may be treated to allow better function of the vocal folds.

Treatment for Vocal Fold Paralysis/Paresis/Fixation

During the initial post-operative days, no treatment is recommended. In many cases, recovery time is all that's needed before full return of function is noted. In cases where voice changes persist after a week, typically a laryngeal stroboscopic examination will be conducted. This examination is conducted using a high definition endoscope with a strobe light through the mouth that allows for a magnified image of the larynx. This examination allows the SLP to determine the extent of the vocal fold paralysis and determine appropriate treatment options.

Voice Therapy

In some cases, voice therapy may be recommended. The goal of therapy will be to improve the closure of the vocal folds and, in doing so, the quality of your voice as well. This therapy usually only requires 3-4 sessions and home practice exercises. Improvement in voicing can often be seen after the first session.

Vocal Fold Augmentation

Voice therapy, however, is only recommended in the presence of a mild problem with vocal fold closure. A more significant issue will not likely resolve with therapy. In these cases, vocal fold *augmentation* may be recommended. This involves an injection into the affected vocal fold using a "filler" material approved for this purpose. The injection serves to increase the size of the paralyzed vocal fold and fill in a portion of the "gap" during vocal fold closure/voicing. This allows the unaffected vocal fold to now make contact with the paralyzed side, improving the voicing ability.

Augmentation injections can be temporary or long-lasting in nature, depending on the nature of the paralysis. If the nerve damage is expected to improve, a temporary injection will be performed. In this case, the material breaks down over time and typically only lasts 2-3 months. During the 2-3 months following injection, a patient is able to have a more normal vocal quality during the nerve recovery period. Because, the effect of the injection is only temporary, it allows for return of normal nerve function without a permanent affect on the affected vocal fold. A temporary injection can be performed repeatedly, if needed, until normal function returns. If nerve function has not returned at one year post-injury, it is considered a permanent impairment and a long-term treatment can be performed at that time.

Medialization Thyroplasty

In some more rare cases, the gap between the vocal folds during voicing is too large for an injection to be effective. In this case, a *medialization thyroplasty* may be advised. This procedure places an implant alongside the paralyzed vocal fold and served to push it toward the center of the larynx where the other vocal fold will be able to close against it for voicing. This procedure is only used in cases where the nerve impairment is permanent and the gap between the vocal folds is too great to "fix" with an augmentation injection alone. In some cases, the thyroplasty will be conducted in combination with an augmentation injection to provide the best possible outcome.

After a thorough stroboscopic examination, you SLP will be able to determine the most appropriate treatment plan to improve voicing. A combination of treatments may produce the best outcome and your SLP and physician will work in close collaboration to ensure the best voice is achieved following treatment.

Potential Radiation Changes to Vocal Cords/Larynx

For cancers involving the vocal cords, radiation effects to the voice are typically far more significant than for radiation patients not affected by larynx cancer. As the neck is a radiation target for head & neck cancers of all types, the vocal cords/larynx may still be affected but to a lesser extent.

Laryngeal Webbing

This is most often seen in cancers directly involving the larynx. In this case, the vocal cords develop scarring that extends *between* the vocal cords; in essence, fusing them together much like webbing on a duck's foot. Depending on the severity of the webbing, it may or may not change the voice significantly. Cases of webbing involving $\geq 1/3$ vocal cords will usually have associated voice changes. With very large webbing, there may even be a reduction in the airway as the vocal cords sit at the upper end of the trachea, although this is more rare in nature.

Treatment for Webbing

In most cases, no surgical treatment for laryngeal webbing is advised unless the webbing is severe in nature and presenting an airway issue. Surgery involving the vocal cords can lead to additional scarring and may not be successful in improving vocal quality. For this reason, optimizing the voice through therapy is typically the preferred treatment.

Radiation Fibrosis

Fibrosis can be thought of as a type of scar tissue that develops between the healthy tissues of the larynx. In the vocal colds, this can result in stiffness that doesn't allow them to vibrate well. In some cases, it can even prevent them from coming together completely. This is the most common reason for voice changes following radiation for head & neck cancer. Patients experiencing fibrosis effects to the voice may notice a deeper voice, a higher-pitch voice, breathiness and/or generalized hoarseness.

Fibrosis effects every patient very differently and to a different extent. Because fibrosis is considered a *latent* effect of radiation, voice changes may evolve gradually over time and become worse over several months.

Treatment for Radiation Fibrosis

There is no surgery to help the fibrosis effects to the larynx in most cases. Voice therapy can usually help and result in improved elasticity and flexibility of the vocal cords. Although the voice may never return to "normal," therapy can usually help improve tone, loudness and pitch range. Your SLP can guide you in realistic expectations regarding your voice following radiation.

Radiation Scarring

The vocal cords are comprised of *layers* that surround a muscle. These layers are comprised of different types of cells, including a fluid-filled layer that assists with the smooth vibration of the vocal cords. Radiation can create scarring in the vocal cords that serves to fuse these layers to each other. In some cases, this scarring may only impact a portion of the vocal cord, but in other cases the scarring is extensive and affects the entire vocal cord.

Changes to the voice from scarring are very similar to changes seen with fibrosis. Similarly, scarring is a latent affect from radiation and the voice may deteriorate over time following completion of radiation treatment.

Treatment for Radiation Scarring

In some cases, surgical intervention for scarring may be indicated although these are generally in the most severe cases as additional surgery to the vocal folds can add to scarring effects. In most cases, no surgical intervention is warranted and patient will be best served through voice therapy designed to optimize their vocal quality. As the scarring cannot be reversed, a return to "normal" may not be realistic. Through therapy, however, pitch, quality and loudness may be improved.

Vocal Hygeine: Caring for your Voice

Taking care of your voice will always be important, especially following radiation treatment for head & neck cancer. Proper voice care or *vocal hygiene* will ensure you have the best voice possible. Also understanding the capacity and limitations of your voice following treatment will help you to manage your voice use and demands to best serve your needs. Your SLP can discuss your individual capacities following treatment. Should you have any questions about your voice care, you should always ask your SLP.

Vocal Hygiene Protocol

Regardless of the cause of your voice disorder or the management plan prescribed, good vocal hygiene is always advised. Taking care of your voice in the best way possible will ensure optimal outcomes and ensure that you maintain your quality voice over time.

In doing so, it is important to remember the following guidelines:

- Drink plenty of non-caffeinated, non-alcoholic fluids (64 oz/day)
-
- Avoid caffeine
-
- Avoid alcohol
-
- DON'T SMOKE or use other tobacco products
-
- Avoid smoky environments such as bars
-
- Avoid Shouting/Yelling
-
- Do not raise your voice louder than normal conversational loudness
  - Instead of yelling up/down the stairs, use your feet, -and a normal loudness.
  - Don't try to compete with noise: turn the volume down on televisions and radios before you try to talk to someone.
  - Avoid talking on the phone in the car
  - Try not to talk over loud freeway/outdoor noise
  - Avoid noisy restaurants and bars
-
- **Give your voice a rest at the end of the day (after 5pm)**
  - Engage in activities that don't involve talking: reading, watching tv, etc.
  - Try to make all your phone calls before 5pm

- - Try not to answer the phone after 5pm, "let the machine get it."
  - Use email/texting as much as possible after 5pm to assist with resting your voice

-
- Avoid throat drops or anything with menthol/eucalyptus (these are very irritating to the larynx)

-
- Use hard candies (regular or sugar free) to keep your throat lubricated if desired. (Avoid mint, sour candies)

-
- Don't whisper if your voice is bad: hoarseness can be a sign your voice needs a break! Limit talking and write instead.

Tracheostomy

A tracheostomy serves to provide an alternate airway, or breathing passage, through the neck, instead of the typical route through the nose and mouth. Although there are various reasons why a tracheotomy may be conducted, in each case, it will allow for respiration through the neck.

Indications

The most common reason a tracheostomy is used in head & neck cancer patients is to provide an alternate airway when the upper airway (passageways of the throat and mouth) is not sufficiently *patent* (open) and may restrict or entirely block the patient's ability to breath. For this reason, a tracheostomy may be used for short periods of time, such as during the acute post-operative phase when swelling may be an issue. Additionally, a tracheostomy may be used on a more long-term basis when there are persistent (long-standing) changes to the upper airway that will restrict the flow of air.

Another indication for tracheostomy may be to ensure the pulmonary health of a patient with severe swallowing difficulty. In this case, saliva or other material that may not be properly swallowed may be suctioned from the trachea to maintain lung health.

Tracheotomy vs Tracheostomy

Although these terms are often used interchangeably, *tracheotomy* refers to the actual surgical procedure involved in creating a *tracheostomy*, or opening in the trachea (windpipe), through which breathing is then possible.

Tracheotomy Procedure

The tracheotomy surgery is a relatively simple procedure during which a cut is made between the cartilage rings of the upper trachea. Once an incision is made and secured, a tracheostomy tube is inserted. During respiration, airflow is then diverted through the tracheostomy tube, bypassing the respiratory passages of the throat, mouth and nose.

Trach Tube Anatomy 101

Although several varieties of tracheostomy tubes exist, the general anatomy remains the same. Some specialty or custom tubes may have different/alternate features, the general "anatomy" of the tube is essentially the same.

Face Plate

This is the "collar" of the trach tube, to which the ties or sutures are connected to secure the tube in place. On this you will see numbers and letters that tell your healthcare provider what kind of trach tube you have in place as well as the dimensions of the tube.

Outer Cannula

Most tubes have an "outer" and an "inner" tube or *cannula.* The outer cannula is connected to the face plate and stays in place until it is time for your tube to be replaced. The width, or diameter, of the outer cannula takes up space in your trachea. If the outer cannula diameter (O.D.) is too large in comparison with your trachea, there may be difficulty using certain speaking valves.

Inner Cannula

The inner cannula sits inside the outer cannula and is designed to be removed and cleaned or removed and replaced. As mucous builds up within the inner cannula (normal) the airway is narrowed. By removing the inner cannula, the airway is improved as the patient is able to breath freely through the space of the outer cannula. This is especially important in the event of a mucous plug that may block the entire inner cannula. The resulting inability to breath is quickly corrected by removing the inner cannula.

Shaft

This refers to the portion of the tube *behind* the face plate. In other words, the part of the tube that is inside the body. Standard adult tracheostomy tubes are typically ~75mm in length which is generally sufficient for most adults. For necks that may be thicker in diameter, longer tracheostomy tubes are available. This means the shaft will be longer than the standard, however, the portion of the tube in front of the face plate is usually the same length as a standard tube.

Curvature

The curvature of the tube refers to the area where there is a bend in the shaft. The curvature is generally standardized across tubes although custom tubes may be ordered to accommodate a different location and/or angle of curvature. There are some tubes that are flexible as well, allowing the tube to curve according to the patient's anatomy.

The curvature is an important feature of the tracheostomy tube. In order to be effective, the tube must be rigid enough to maintain an open airway. It's also important that the shaft of the tube not come in contact with the trachea once it passes through the tracheotomy site. The tissues of the trachea are somewhat delicate and direct contact with the trach tube may result in injury/trauma to the trachea.

The curvature is specified so that the shaft of the tube passes essentially horizontally through the soft tissues of the neck, enters the trachea, and the curvature should ensure the shaft of the tube is "floating" within the trachea. Like a tube within a tube. If the curvature is not appropriate for the patient, the tube may then rest or even push against the trachea, likely causing damage.

Cuff

Not every tube has a cuff. The *cuff* of a tracheostomy tube is a balloon-like structure attached to the outer cannula below the level of the curvature. A cuff can be inflated with air to fill the space in the trachea between the tracheal wall and the outer cannula. When a cuff is not needed, however, it can be deflated as well. There are various types of coughs as well as reasons for using cuffed tracheostomy tubes. For more information on the use of cuffed trach tubes, see "Cuffed vs. Cuffless Tubes" (below).

Pilot Balloon

This feature is only found on a cuffed tube. It is a small plastic balloon with a valve seal that is attached to the shaft of the balloon by a lead line. The pilot balloon lead line is usually attached to the outer cannula near the face plate. The cuff is inflated and deflated via this balloon and the status of the cuff inflation can also be determined fairly well by the inflation status of the pilot balloon. Since the cuff itself sits deep within the trachea, it is impossible to see the cuff status directly. However, if the pilot balloon is inflated, this is an indication the cuff is inflated as well. Similarly, if the balloon is flat, or deflated, this is an indication the cuff is likely deflated.

Although the pilot balloon is an indication regarding the status of the cuff, it is impossible to determine the exact degree of inflation vs deflation based on the pilot balloon alone. For more information regarding cuff status, see "Assessing Cuff Status" (below).

Fenestration(s)

A *fenestration* is a hole in the shaft of the tracheostomy tube, above the curvature, and therefore also above the cuff of a cuffed trach tube. The purpose of a fenestration is to allow for airflow upward and through the vocal cords. Without airflow through the vocal cords, a tracheostomy patient will not be able to produce a voice.

A fenestration is not necessary to be able to talk with a tracheostomy tube, although it will likely improve the loudness and ease of producing a voice. For more information, see Speaking with a Tracheostomy Tube below.

On a fenestrated tube, there is a fenestration in the outer cannula. In order for the fenestration to be of any benefit for voicing, however, the inner cannula must also be fenestrated.

There are advantages and disadvantages to fenestrated tubes. More information on this topic can be found in Pros and Cons of Tube Fenestrations below.

Tracheostomy Tube Varieties

There are a variety of tracheostomy tubes available. The doctor will determine which is the most appropriate based on individual health factors and needs. Below are descriptions of the most common varieties but custom tubes are also used when traditional options are not sufficient to meet the needs of unique patients.

Cuffed vs Cuffless Tubes

A "cuff" refers to a balloon type structure located around the outer cannula, below the curvature, at the upper portion of the lower 1/3 of the tracheostomy tube and can be inflated and deflated as needed. A cuff can be inflated with air to fill the space in the trachea between the tracheal wall and the outer cannula which is necessary for various reasons/conditions.

Standard tracheostomy tube are designed as "cuffed" or "cuffless" and your doctor will decide which tube is most appropriate for you.

Cuffed tubes are most often used during mechanical ventilation. In this case, the cuff seals the airway so that the breaths being delivered by the ventilator (respirator) are delivered directly to the lungs. Without proper cuff inflation, the delivered breath (or a portion of it) would escape around the tube and out the nose and mouth without going to the lungs.

Cuffs can also be inflated to help protect the airway and lungs from foreign material. For example, if a patient is unable to swallow their saliva properly, these secretions may overflow in the throat and enter the windpipe, resulting in "aspiration." Even aspiration of saliva has the potential to make someone very sick because of the bacteria it introduces to the sterile lungs. In this case, a cuffed tube may be indicated. With proper inflation of the cuff ("sealing the trachea"), the lungs are better protected from the saliva.

Types of Cuffs

High Volume/Low Pressure

This is the most common cuff found on a standard tracheostomy tube. These cuffs have a larger structure and, in turn, surface area against the trachea, using a higher volume of air to inflate the "balloon." In this sense, the contact area against the trachea is larger, allowing the potential for a better seal. Similarly, because of the high volume of the balloon and greater surface contact against the trachea, an effective seal can be established without a great deal of pressure against the trachea.

The drawback to this form of cuff also pertains to the larger size of the "balloon." Even when entirely deflated, the shell of the cuff fills the trachea to some extent. Consider a grape vs a raisin. An inflated cuff is like the grape. The air in a cuff is like the water in a grape. Although a raisin is smaller than the grape, it still has a volume. The same is true of the cuff. It may "shrivel" once the air if removed, but it still occupies space in the trachea, more than just the tube shaft itself.

When weaning from a tracheostomy tube or when using a speaking valve, the extra volume of a deflated high volume/low pressure cuff may have a negative impact on the expected outcomes.

Low Volume/High Pressure

In general, these cuffs are not ideal for patients requiring long-term use of a cuff. These cuffs typically conform to the shaft of the tube, expanding when air is inflated under high pressure.

The benefit of these cuffs is that the tube can act essentially as a cuffless tube, although has the potential for cuff inflation when needed. However, since these are high pressure inflations, the surface pressure against the tracheal wall is also quite high and may present a risk for tissue damage if used over a prolonged period of time.

So why these cuffs? Unlike the high volume/low pressure cuff, there is no residual space taken up in the trachea when this cuff is deflated. In most cases, with full deflation, this cuff will adhere to the shaft of the tube.

In some cases, then, this type of cuff can be ideal. For example, consider a tracheostomy patient. not ordinarily needing cuff inflation, however, may need to undergo one or more future procedures under anesthesia. Since a cuff is required to maintain adequate ventilation while under anesthesia, this presents and ideal situation. The patient can experience the benefits of a cuffless trach, although no tube change will be required for general anesthesia as the cuff can be inflated for the procedure (short-term), and then deflated for normal breathing/speaking.

Proper Cuff Inflation

The trachea is a sensitive structure and like any part of the body, relies on adequate blood flow for proper tissue health and function. If too much pressure is applied to the trachea, again like any other portion of the body, blood flow to this are will be restricted or even cut off entirely. When this happens, the tissues begin to deteriorate and may even die.

When discussing cuff inflation then, it is important to understand this principle. The purpose of the cuff inflation is to seal the airway. Yet too much pressure against the trachea may cause damage to these tissues. This is why proper cuff inflation is important.

To inflate a cuff, a syringe filled with air is connected to the pilot balloon. Once properly connected, the air is the pushed into the cuff with the syringe.

Proper cuff inflation occurs when the cuff effectively seals the airway, while also exerting the least amount of necessary pressure against the trachea. Since every person is different, there is no safe "standard" to use for every patient regarding how much air to use during cuff inflation. General guidelines apply but your doctor will use various methods to determine how much air results in appropriate cuff inflation.

Assessing Cuff Status

The pilot balloon will always be the best guide for helping to determine if a cuff is inflated, deflated, or somewhere in-between. If the balloon is flat, one can assume the cuff is largely deflated. If it is "puffy," some level of inflation exists. For adequate cuff inflation however, the pilot balloon is merely a guide; typical manometry measurements of cuff pressures are far more reliable to determine cuff status.

Manometry measurement is also very helpful in determining if there may be a leak in the cuff (similar to a leak in a tire or a balloon). If a patient requires cuff inflation, a leak in the cuff will not allow for adequate use. In this case, the tracheostomy tube should be replaced.

Fenestrated vs. Non-Fenestrated Tubes

A *fenestration* is a hole in the shaft of the tracheostomy tube, above the curvature, and therefore also above the cuff of a cuffed trach tube. The purpose of a fenestration is to allow for airflow upward and through the vocal cords. Without airflow through the vocal cords, a tracheostomy patient will not be able to produce a voice.

A fenestration is not necessary to be able to talk with a tracheostomy tube, although it will likely improve the loudness and ease of producing a voice. Although a fenestrated tube can make speech much easier for tracheostomy patients, it is important to understand that you **must** use a fenestrated inner cannula as well to achieve the benefits of the fenestration. Standard, non-fenestrated inner cannulas (most common) will block the fenestration, thus blocking the airflow benefits as well.

Although a fenestration can have benefits for speaking, there are also some other factors to consider when determining if a fenestrated tube should be used. Because the fenestration is typically aligned along the curved portion of the shaft, there is a potential the fenestration will contact the tracheal wall. If this occurs, the edge of the fenestration may produced contact irritation and trauma to the tracheal lining. In some cases, this can result in the development of a *granuloma.* A granuloma is a reactive tissue formation (like a blister or callous) that can have a bulbous or ball-like shape. These are highly vascularized, can bleed easily and may interfere with inner cannula removal/replacement. As long as there is continued irritation, the granuloma is likely to stay and even grow.

When granulomas develop in reaction to the fenestration contact, they will generally grow through the fenestration and into the lumen of the tube shaft. As this happens, there may be limitations to airflow, as the granuloma is now obstructing the clear flow of air through the tube. In this way also, the patient achieves no benefit from the fenestration since the space is now blocked by granuloma tissue. The granuloma will also make it difficult for the tube to be removed as it grows through the fenestration.

Simple endoscopic examination *through* the tracheostomy tube will determine if there is granuloma formation, although there are other indications patients are able to identify themselves. For example, if the granuloma is growing through the fenestration, removal and reinsertion of the inner cannula may become more difficult. There may also be notable bleeding with inner cannula changes. Granulomas are filled with a great deal of small, fragile blood vessels. Because of this, they are very prone to bleeding. When changing an inner cannula, there should normally be no contact with tracheal tissue. For this reason, if you notice even small amounts of blood during or after inner cannula changes, you should mention this to your doctor for further evaluation.

Although granulomas are not worrisome in nature, they can contribute to complications that can be difficult to manage. If you are concerned in this regard, your doctor or SLP staff can examine you further.

Use of a fenestrated tube is generally not recommended when cuff inflation is required to protect the airway from aspiration. Since the fenestration is located above the cuff, saliva and secretions can fall through the fenestration, limiting this benefit of cuff inflation. It is important to remember, however, that a fenestrated tube can have the same benefit in this regard as a non-fenestrated tube, simply by using a non-fenestrated inner cannula.

Your doctor will always determine which tube is the most appropriate for you, but understanding tube principles can help you better manage and maintain your tracheostomy.

Being a "Neck Breather"

Once a tracheostomy is in place, respiration is occurring (mostly) through the tracheostomy tube. Although the upper respiratory passageways are still connected to the trachea and lungs, airflow will always follow basic laws of physics, in this case: the path of least resistance.

It will always be easier for airflow to travel through the open tracheostomy tube than through the passageways of the throat, mouth and nose. For this reason, a patient with a tracheostomy is known as a "neck breather."

This is an important distinction! Since the majority of the air you breath will pass through the neck, it also means it is *not* passing through the nose and mouth. There are some significant changes that occur as a result.

Physiologic/Functional Changes

Smelling

Following a tracheostomy, many patients report not being able to smell as they did before. The sense of smell, or *olfaction*, remains intact as there is no impact from the surgery to the nerves of olfaction that allow for smelling scents, aromas and odors. What *has* changed, however, is the pathway of airflow during respiration. Prior to the tracheostomy, air would flow into the body through the nose and mouth. This movement of air through the nose allowed for scents and aromas to be detected as the smells came in contact with the tiny nerve endings in the nose that are responsible for the sense of smell.

Following a tracheostomy, however, there is minimal, if any, active flow of air through the nose during breathing. This can be perceived as a loss of smell. Olfaction can be restored, at least temporarily, by covering the end of the tracheostomy tube and allowing air to be inhaled through the nose. For short instances (example: smelling a rose), this can help a tracheostomy patient better appreciate scents and aromas. This technique, however, may not be comfortable (or even possible) if the upper passageways of respiration are severely blocked.

Tasting

Because our sense of taste is strongly related to our sense of smell, you will notice that foods may no longer taste the way they did before the surgery. The tongue is able to detect five basic tastes: sweet, sour, salt, bitter and savory. ~70% of our sense of taste, however, comes from our sense of smell. Our sense of smell adds to the taste of our food and allows us to recognize the difference between steak and pizza, for example. Once you start eating following a tracheostomy, you will notice that your favorite foods may taste quite different from what you remember.

Coughing

Coughing as a neck breather means anything you should expel from your lungs will be expelled or coughed out through your stoma. Although you are accustomed to covering your mouth when you cough, you will learn instead to cover your tube opening. Initially following surgery and for several weeks thereafter, you will likely cough a great deal of mucous and secretions from your lungs. The lungs are increasing the output of secretions and mucous in response to the changes in your anatomy and physiology. Regular application of an HME assists with restoring normal lung function by delivering the heated/warmed and humidified air the lungs are accustomed to. Over time with regular IIME application, the secretion production will slow down.

Many patients are concerned to see, despite regular HME application, they continue to cough mucous from their tube. It should be stressed that the lungs should normally produce mucous in healthy people as a protective layer to help keep lung tissue moist as well as to serve to trap inhaled particles that may be harmful to lung tissue. In any person, these secretions are coughed frequently during the course of a normal day and typically swallowed. Following a tracheostomy, however, these secretions must be expelled from the tube and wiped away.

Filtration

Before a tracheostomy, the nose helps to filter the air that is inhaled. After the surgery, all the air you breathe goes in and out of the tracheostomy tube, bypassing the natural filtration of the nose. It is very important to stay away from smoke, dust and other pollutants, as these will be inhaled directly into your lungs.

Humidification

The air we inhale, is typically filtered, heated and humidified first as it passes through the moist pathway of the nose, mouth and throat. Following a tracheostomy, however, this is no longer the case. As a result, the air that is inhaled directly by the lungs is less humid than is normal. This can result in changes to lung function and secretion management. For this reason, we will always recommend methods to improve the humidification of the lung tissues and passageways. The following details various options used in this practice. These can be used alone or in combination with one another. Your doctor/SLP staff will inform you of the most appropriate way to compensate for diminished humidification.

HMEs: In addition to filtering the air, breathing in through the nose and mouth also helps to heat and humidify air that is inhaled. After a tracheostomy, inhaled air through the tube enters the lungs without first being humidified or heated since it is no longer being inhaled through the nose/mouth. A heat and moisture exchange cap, or HME, can be utilized after your surgery to assist with these changes.

Electric Humidifiers: It is also recommended by this practice that patients begin using humidifiers, especially at night by the bedside. Regular inhalation of non-humidified air can have a drying effect on the tissues of the respiratory tract and lungs. Breathing non-humidified air will also cause thickening and drying of lung secretions/mucous and contribute to the formation of mucous plugs. A mucous plug is a collection of thickened mucous that is large enough to potentially plug the tracheostomy tube. Proper humidification can assist in minimizing the potential for developing mucous plugs.

Sterile Saline: A saline bullet is a term used to describe a small vial of sterile saline. These can range in size from 5-30ml. The small, sterile packaging makes them easy to use for travel purposes.

Saline is used to provide quick, temporary moisture to the pulmonary air passages and lungs and are most commonly used to correct issues related to inadequate humidification for tracheostomy patients not regularly using HMEs.

Saline bullet utilization can be helpful in loosening dried mucous and mucous plugs as well as restoring moisture to dry airways. These should only be used on the advice of your doctor or SLP staff.

Tracheostomy patients using an HME typically will not need saline bullets once their HME use is initiated and consistent.

Speaking

Following a tracheostomy, the airflow during normal breathing is diverted through the tube, which sits below the vocal cords in the throat. As a result, air will no longer be able to flow through the vocal cords. Although the larynx (voice box) and vocal cords are not affected by the tracheostomy, the loss of airflow through the vocal cords will prevent normal voice/speech production. There are, however, ways to restore speech in a tracheostomy patient. For more information on this, see Speaking with a Tracheostomy Tube below.

Swallowing

Many patients are able to swallow very well following a tracheostomy. There are, however, physiologic and mechanical changes that occur with a tracheostomy that can result in swallowing impairment. Your SLP is extremely knowledgeable in assisting patients with swallowing following a tracheostomy. For more information on this topic see Swallowing with a Tracheostomy (below).

Speaking with a Tracheostomy Tube

Understanding How a Voice is Produced

The vocal cords, of course are very important in producing a voice. They are positioned at the top of the *trachea*, or windpipe, and have the ability to open and close. When we breathe, the vocal cords are open, but they come together in order to make a voice or *phonate.* The vocal cords coming together, however, will not result in a voice. In fact, the vocal cords *do not vibrate independently*. In order to produce a voice, the vocal cords must come together, while *simultaneously*, air from the lungs is exhaled through them in a sufficient manner. The flow of air through the closed vocal cords produces voicing.

Following a tracheostomy, the airflow during normal breathing is diverted through the tube, which sits below the vocal cords in the throat. As a result, air will no longer be able to flow through the vocal cords. Although the larynx (voice box) and vocal cords are not affected by the tracheostomy, the loss of airflow through the vocal cords will prevent normal voice/speech production. There are, however, ways to restore speech in a tracheostomy patient. Your doctor/SLP staff will determine the most appropriate method for you.

DEFLATE THE CUFF!!!

For the methods described here, any cuff must be deflated, -as much as possible. Even a deflated cuff can take up space in the airway, limiting the airflow available to speak. Because of this, it's best to deflate the cuff as much as possible.

Finger Occlusion

For tracheostomy patients, the finger occlusion technique is the quickest, easiest and least expensive way to restore speech. For this method, simply use your finger to seal the end of the tube when you want to talk. This will divert the air through the vocal cords (instead of exiting out the tube). After speaking, remove your finger to allow for normal breathing through the tracheostomy.

This technique, however, should only be used when the hands are clean as bacteria can easily be introduced from the fingers to the tube, presenting a potential for infecting the airway and lungs.

Speaking Valves

Speaking valves are the most common method of restoring voice following a tracheostomy. These may also be used in-line with a ventilator in some cases. Although a speaking valve provides excellent voice restoration, these valves are not appropriate for all patients. Your doctor/SLP staff will determine if you are a candidate for a speaking valve and select the most appropriate valve for you. In this practice, there are two main types of speaking valves prescribed/utilized.

Passy-Muir Speaking Valve (PMV)

The PMV is a speaking valve placed as a cap, over the end of the tracheostomy tube. There are various versions, although the technical function is the same across valves.

The PMV is the most commonly used speaking valve in this practice for the many benefits its "positive closure" design offers. Although other speaking valves exist, this is the only one with the "positive closure" feature. The "positive closure" valve means that the valve *remains closed* until a sufficient amount of inhalation pressure is applied. In contrast, other speaking valves close in response to exhaled air pressure, otherwise they remain open to some degree. There are several benefits to the positive closure design for head & neck cancer patients.

Of course, the primary benefit from this valve is restoring speech to the tracheostomy patient. By remaining closed, the valve redirects exhaled air upward through the vocal cords automatically. No extra time/effort/airflow is required to close the valve.

Because the valve remains in a closed position, except during active inhalation, all cough efforts are directed through the throat and mouth, more similar to normal physiologic function in this regard. This design also helps ensure no air is lost through the tube, leaving the patient able to more effectively cough since there is more air available.

The positive closure feature also means secretions are prevented from entering the tube or the speaking valve which can mean less cleaning and more reliable function as a result.

Swallowing and the PMV

The closing of the vocal cords also plays a very important role in the swallow process. By closing during the swallow, the vocal cords prevent any air from leaving the lungs during the swallow. This *subglottic pressure* is important for driving a strong swallow.

In a tracheostomy patient, even if the vocal cords close as they should during the swallow, the typical subglottic pressurization is not achieved since the open tracheostomy tube is creating an opening for air to leave the lungs. As such, it is not uncommon to experience a degree of swallowing difficulty following a tracheostomy.

The PMV, however, because it remains in a closed position during swallowing, allows for subglottic pressure to be maintained, thus helping to restore normal physiology for swallowing. For this reason, in particular, this valve is typically used over other speaking valve options.

It can be difficult for head & neck cancer patients to safely tolerate a PMV. Because the valve remains closed except during inhalation, the patient must be able to effectively exhale through the passageways of the nose and mouth. For this reason, it may not be appropriate for certain patients. Your doctor/SLP staff can answer any further questions you may have in this regard.

Shikani Speaking Valve

Although the PMV is preferred for its positive closure design, for those patients that are unable to tolerate it, the Shikani Speaking Valve may provide a viable option, especially for the head & neck cancer patients.

This valve is designed with a small plastic ball that forms the valve and the valve itself can be configured different ways to allow for more easy breathing through the tube vs easier valve closure for talking. As a result, this valve design can be better tolerated by those patients who are unable to breath comfortably with the PMV.

Specialty Tubes

There are certain tracheostomy tubes designed with the sole purpose of allowing for oral speech when more traditional options are not possible. Your SLP will work with you to ensure your optimal communication/swallowing status and can discuss the potential benefits of these tube options as appropriate. Typically speaking, however, the vast majority of patients can achieve a functional communication status without the need of a specialty tube for this purpose.

Swallowing with a Tracheostomy

Many patients reports changes in their swallowing following a tracheostomy. Although many patients swallow very well following a tracheostomy, there are several factors why a change in swallowing may be noticed.

For this reason, should you notice any changes in your swallow ability, or begin coughing, choking during eating, it is extremely important to notify your doctor/SLP. Following an evaluation, your SLP be able to better manage your swallowing for the best function possible.

If at any time you notice food/drink material being coughed and expelled from the tracheostomy tube, you should always contact your doctor and/or SLP immediately. This may be an indication of a swallowing problem that could have very severe health implications.

Subglottic Pressurization

The closing of the vocal cords also plays a very important role in the swallow process. By closing during the swallow, the vocal cords prevent any air from leaving the lungs during the swallow. This *subglottic pressure* is important for driving a strong swallow.

In a tracheostomy patient, even if the vocal cords *adduct* (close) as they should during the swallow, the typical subglottic pressurization is not achieved since the open tracheostomy tube is creating an opening for air to leave the lungs. As such, many patients may experience swallowing difficulty following their tracheostomy.

A Passy-Muir Speaking Valve (PMV) can be utilized to assist with swallowing difficulties when subglottic pressurization appears to be a contributing factor. For this reason, if you have been provided with a PMV, it is always recommended you are wearing the valve during meals, but also as often as possible, while awake, is ideal in this regard, as it will also help with the regular swallowing of saliva and other secretions throughout the day.

Hyolaryngeal Movement

During a normal swallow, the larynx (voice box), along with other attached muscles/structures, moves upward and outward. This is referred to as *hyolaryngeal movement* and can be observed when you watch or feel your Adam's apple (thyroid cartilage) move up and down during a swallow.

In normal human anatomy, the larynx is attached to the trachea, through which the tracheostomy tube has been inserted and rests following a tracheostomy. In some cases, the tube can contribute to less hyolaryngeal movement as a result. Any changes in swallowing following a tracheostomy should always be reported to your doctor and/or SLP staff. Although the tracheostomy may not be contributing to any perceived swallowing problem, proper evaluation of the swallow function should be conducted to ensure the patient is eating as safely and effectively as possible.

Suction

Most tracheostomy patients are prescribed a suction machine when returning home following surgery. Use of the suction will be helpful in removing mucous and other secretions from the tube, ensuring a clear airway.

Despite having a suction machine, it is important to use a *simultaneous* strong cough. Without strong and forceful coughs, mucous will not be cleared adequately from lower portions of the airways.

Many patients find it helpful to use saline bullets to assist with clearing/suctioning of their secretions. Use of saline bullets can significantly help to thin the secretions while also moisturizing the airways. In this sense, coughing/suctioning can be much easier. If you find it is difficult to clear your mucous/secretions from your tracheostomy tube, even with using suction, it may be helpful to use saline bullets to assist in this regard. Your doctor or SLP staff can discuss this further with you.

Because the tracheostomy now provides a direct pathway into the lungs, it is important to always keep your suction components as clean as possible. Emptying the canister regularly as well as changing the suction tubing/attachments according to the manufacturer's recommendations is extremely important in this regard.

Although various suction machines exist, regardless of the model you are provided with, instructions for proper care and operation will always be included. Once you read through these, your SLP can assist you in a better understanding if needed.

Generally speaking, however, the tip of the suction, can serve as a way of introducing bacteria into your tracheostomy tube. Although your tube is not a sterile environment, keeping the tube and suction as clean as possible will help to minimize the potential for bacteria/viruses from entering the lungs this way. Whether you are using a Yankouer tip or suction catheter, you should never allow the tip of your suction (the part you touch the tracheostomy tube with), to come in contact with soiled surfaces. Placing the tip in a clean sandwich bag or glass can help ensure it is somewhat protected between uses. Never use the suction if the tip (Yankouer/catheter) is visibly dirty or touches the floor/other similarly soiled surfaces without first properly cleaning or even replacing if adequate cleaning is not possible.

Tracheostomy Care

To ensure adequate function of the tracheostomy, and to minimize potential complications from the tracheostomy, proper care and maintenance is important.

Tracheostomy Site
Typical wound care instructions will apply during the initial days following a tracheotomy. Application of an antibacterial agent will typically be prescribed by your surgeon to use over the initial post-operative days. There will be a small amount of blood/bloody drainage during these initial days as well, which is normal. Should there be signs of infection, however, you should contact your doctor immediately.

Potential Signs of Infection
Typical signs of infection would be worsening/intense pain at the wound site after the first 2-3 days. Typically, pain associated with a tracheotomy is not severe and should improve over the first 3-5 days following surgery. If this does not happen, however, it is important to contact your physician for further evaluation.

Any significant swelling/ inflammation, especially an increase after the first four post-operative days, may be an indication of a local infection and should be reported to your doctor. Although it may be difficult and/or uncomfortable to use tracheostomy ties in the presence of significant selling, it is important that the tube be properly secured. Ties that are too loose or left untied can allow the tracheostomy tube to come out entirely. Never leave a tube unsecured.

Any drainage or discharge from the wound should be clear. Thicker or more opaque secretions (like puss) should be reported to your doctor. Also, a foul smell not previously noted may be an indication of infection or other issue and should also be reported.

Cleaning

Prior to discharge from the hospital following your tracheotomy, nursing staff should provide you with care/cleaning instructions. Daily cleaning of your tube is important, which may include cleaning and/or replacing the inner cannula. There are commercially available tracheostomy cleaning kits available which are very helpful in helping with the care of your tracheostomy.

Following the manufacturer's guidelines for cleaning is important. Always ask your nurse of doctor for proper care instructions as these may vary depending on the tracheostomy tube you have.

Decannulation

Decannulation refers to the removal of the tracheostomy tube once it is no longer required. Your doctor will determine when decannulation is appropriate and this can be conducted very easily in the office.

Before it is determined that you no longer require your tracheostomy tube, your doctor may conduct trials to determine how you tolerate breathing through the nose and mouth again. There trials are usually done via two methods: *weaning* or *capping.* Often times, capping will be conducted at the end of a weaning trial to ensure you are ready to return to breathing through your upper respiratory tract.

Weaning

This process can be conducted various ways, although the most common is to begin by using a Passy-Muir Speaking Valve (PMV) if you are not already using one. The PMV requires you to exhale through the nose/mouth while still allowing you to inhale via the tracheostomy tube. In this sense, you breathe only partially through the tube which serves as a good determinant is assessing if you may be ready to be decannulated. Although not always, if you are unable to tolerate the PMV during prolonged use throughout the day, it is unlikely you are ready to be decannulated.

In some cases, weaning from your tracheostomy tube may also include *down-sizing;* which means your current tracheostomy tube *size* is exchanged to a smaller size. Essentially, the space you have to breath through your tracheostomy is made smaller, usually requiring more respiration activity through the nose and mouth. Since airflow follows the "path of least resistance," by making the tube size smaller, air should more easily low through the nose and mouth after down-sizing. Although not always, if you are unable to tolerate down-sizing of your tracheostomy tube, it is unlikely you are able to be decannulated.
Down-sizing may be conducted in combination with PMV utilization and/or capping trials during the weaning process.

Capping Trials

Capping trials refers to times when a "cap" is placed over the tracheostomy tube opening to close off airflow via the tube. In doing so, the tube no longer acts as a means of airflow, allowing respiration entirely through the nose and mouth.

Capping trials may be started using a particular schedule, asking you to wear the cap for specified amounts of time. If this is well tolerated, you will be asked to wear the cap 24/7 for a period of a few to several days. If 24/7 capping is well tolerated, this is a good indication the tracheostomy tube is no longer needed and decannulation can be planned.

Although capping trials provide a good sense of how you will tolerate breathing without the tracheostomy tube, it is important to remember that breathing will be easier following decannulation. If the cap is not well tolerated, and no particular upper airway obstruction is noted. It may be that the tube itself is creating too much obstruction to airflow and you may be down-sized as a result. By placing a smaller tube, and replacing a cap, this will allow for improved airflow around the tube and likely, better tolerance for the capping.

Tube Removal and Wound Care

Your doctor will establish how best to assess your ability to breath without a tracheostomy. Although once this is determined, the tracheotomy tube itself is easily removed in the office.

Many patients are surprised to lean the tracheostomy site will close on its own, without requiring suture closure or any additional procedure. In fact, once the tracheostomy tube is removed, the soft tissues of the neck are pressed together and a small dressing is placed over the site. This will close spontaneously over the next few days.

To help ensure quick healing of the trach site, it is very important to apply pressure to the site whenever you cough, talk, swallow and laugh. Without adequate pressure to the site, air will continue to leak from the wound, serving to keep it open instead of allowing it to heal. With consistent pressure during coughing, talking, laughing and swallowing, you will help to allow these tissues to heal more quickly.

As the tracheotomy site will continue to drain for a while, it is important to keep clean, dry dressings in place until the wound site has completely healed. The site itself will heal from the inside out; meaning the trachea will likely close *before* the soft tissues of the neck. While air continues to leak from the site during respiration, speaking, etc., the trachea has not yet closed and particular attention should be pain to ensuring there is adequate manual pressure applied to the wound site when talking and coughing.

Once no further air leakage is noted, it can usually be assumed that the trachea has closed. Although this may happen fairly quickly, the wound site itself may continue to seep/drain slightly for some time. This is very normal as the soft tissues of the neck, outside the trachea, continue to heal.

Accidental Decannulation

Although not common, there is a small possibility the tracheostomy tube may dislodge from the trach site accidentally. In this case, if the tube is clean, an attempt to reinsert it immediately should be made. If you are unable to replace the tube, you should seek immediate attention from an Emergency Department, including calling emeregency medical services if necessary (ambulance/EMT).

Laryngectomy

Anatomical Changes

A laryngectomy is a complex surgery that involves removing the larynx, also known as the "voice box." During this surgery, your surgeon redirects your trachea or "windpipe." A permanent opening, or "stoma" is then created at the front base of your neck. This will be the opening through which you breathe in and out. It is permanent and will not be reversed or closed. The importance of this opening and why it is permanent is often a great concern for patients and will be thoroughly explained in this material. You will also likely have many other questions and concerns. This information is meant to help guide you through a better understanding of the anatomical and physiologic changes it will bring. Please take the time to read this information completely as it will help to answer many common questions and concerns patients and their families have when going into this surgery and recovery process.

Being a "Neck Breather"

In addition to removing the vocal cords, there are other structures that are also parts of your larynx that will be removed. Many of these removed structures are important in swallowing safely and ensuring you do not choke. This explains, when there is a laryngeal cancer, why so many patients find it difficult to eat without choking. Often times, there are diseased parts of the larynx that prevent them from swallowing safely.

When your larynx is removed, including these structures important for safe swallowing, the trachea, or "windpipe" is left open and the food you eat and drink will enter your windpipe and your lungs. For this reason, your windpipe is diverted, or "rerouted," suturing the opening to your neck, disconnecting it from the rest of your throat, and therefore ensuring you will no longer be at risk for choking when you eat.

After your surgery, it is very important that everyone involved in your care understand that you breathe differently from other people. Family members, caregivers and other health professionals should be aware that you no longer can take air in through your nose and mouth. This is very important should you ever need CPR because breaths need to be given through the stoma in your neck or it will not get to your lungs. You should purchase a medical alert bracelet, necklace or lapel pin that states "Neck Breather." It is important that you wear this at all times.

Since you will be breathing through the stoma in your neck, it is also very important that you protect your stoma. Before a laryngectomy, the nose helps to filter the air that is inhaled. After the surgery, all the air you breathe goes in and out of the stoma, bypassing the natural filtration of the nose. It is very important to stay away from smoke, dust and other pollutants as these will be inhaled directly into your lungs.

In addition to filtering the air, breathing in through the nose and mouth also helps to heat and humidify air that is inhaled. After a laryngectomy, inhaled air through the stoma enters the lungs without first being humidified or heated since it is no longer being inhaled through the nose/mouth. A heat and moisture exchange cassette, or HME, will be utilized after your surgery to assist with these changes.

Coughing as a neck breather means anything you should expel from your lungs will be expelled or coughed out through your stoma. Although you are accustomed to covering your mouth when you cough, you will learn instead to cover your stoma. Initially following surgery and for several weeks thereafter, you will cough a great deal of mucous and secretions from your lungs. The lungs are increasing the output of secretions and mucous in response to the changes in your anatomy and physiology. Regular application of the HME assists with restoring normal lung function by delivering the heated/warmed and humidified air the lungs are accustomed to. Over time with regular HME application, the secretion production will slow down.

Many patients are concerned to see, despite regular HME application and sufficient healing from surgery, they continue to cough mucous from their stoma. It should be stressed that that lungs should normally produce mucous in healthy people as a protective layer to help keep lung tissue moist as well as to serve to trap inhaled particles that may be harmful to lung tissue. In a non-laryngectomized patient, these secretions are coughed frequently during the course of a normal day and typically swallowed. Following a laryngectomy, however, these secretions must be expelled from the stoma and wiped away.

Functional Changes

Communication After Surgery

Usually, one of the greatest concerns a laryngectomee patient and family will have relates to communication. The surgery removes the voice box and therefore will take away your ability to speak as you did before. However, modern advancements in voice restoration have allowed laryngectomees to speak with clear, functional and natural sounding voices, often stronger and clearer than before the laryngectomy surgery. What you are able to use to help you speak will depend on the extent of your surgery as well as your recovery.

Immediately after surgery you will need to use non-verbal ways of communicating. It is important for family members, nurses and doctors to ask "yes/no" questions to communicate with you. You may use a blinking method (once=yes; twice=no), or other such techniques to respond. As you begin to recover more, (after a day or so) the Speech Pathologist in the hospital will come to see you and may give you a communication board or a dry-erase board. If you are unable to write for any reason, a communication board will help greatly. With this board, you can point to various word choices as well as spell out words. Once you feel well enough to write, you can use this as a means to communicate everything you may want.

You will soon realize writing is not nearly as efficient in communicating your thoughts as oral speech. For this reason, one of the earliest goals in your rehabilitative process is for you to be an oral communicator again.

An electrolarynx is a device that produces an electronic tone in place of your own voice. This can be used fairly soon after surgery, within a few days, but requires some assistance from a Speech Pathologist to teach you how to use it. Initially this device can be used with a "straw" adapter that is placed in your mouth. Once you begin to heal and the neck is no longer tender, the device is placed on the neck, near the region where your larynx used to be. You will also have to practice a bit so that you can be easily understood. For decades, laryngectomees use this as their primary way of communicating, although with the evolution of the TEP or "tracheoesophageal voice prosthesis, " the electrolarynx is used much less frequently as a primary means of communication. Many successful TEP users, however, will have this as an alternate means of communication as needed or "just in case."

Most patients, however, will be able to speak using the most advanced methods for voice restoration. This is known as tracheoesophageal voice restoration. With this form of voice restoration, a small hole is made in common wall that is shared by the trachea (windpipe) and the esophagus (food pipe). This procedure is typically conducted during your laryngectomy surgery, although can also be completed later as well. A device referred to as a "tracheoesophageal voice prosthesis" or "TEP" is then placed. This device acts as a one-way valve that allows air to pass into the esophagus and flow out of the mouth, but closes when air is not flowing through it to keep food, liquid and saliva out of the trachea.

When using a TEP, voicing is achieved by channeling air from the lungs into the esophagus. Just above the TEP, in the esophagus, and extending into the lower portion of the throat or "pharynx," there is a segment of tissue that vibrates when air passes through it, similarly to how vocal cords vibrate and make a noise. The "voice" this makes is different from your original voice but it gives you a natural sound source that you can now talk with as you did before the surgery. You will need therapy to learn how to use and care for the device but this is relatively short-term in nature. A complete discussion of TEP rehabilitation can be found later in this chapter.

Other Effects of Your Surgery

Because there is no longer any air flowing through the nose after the laryngectomy, you will notice a change in your sense of smell and taste. Your *ability* to smell will be exactly the same as before the surgery in that the nerves, senses and structures involved in smelling will not be changed in any way. Without the flow of air through the nose, however, the capacity to smell changes. In order to smell scents, odors and aromas around us involves having air pass through the nose, carrying small particles into the nose where they are detected by sensory cells in the nose which are then interpreted by the brain and translated into "smells." Since no air will be flowing through the nose after your surgery, it will seem as if you can no longer smell things like you could before. Many laryngectomees find it helpful to use their hand to "waft" air into their nose when they attempt to smell. The speech pathology staff will also teach you a technique which will allow you to draw air through the nasal passages and assist with smelling.

Similarly, because our sense of taste is strongly related to our sense of smell, you will notice that foods may no longer taste the way they did before the surgery. The tongue is able to detect five basic tastes: sweet, sour, salt, bitter and savory. Our sense of smell adds to the taste of our food and allows us to recognize the difference between steak and pizza, for example. Once you start eating after surgery, you will notice that your favorite foods may taste quite different from what you remember.

During SLP visits, you will learn a technique to restore airflow through the nose, allowing you to smell and taste as usual. Many laryngectomees have reported this helps foods taste more "normal." Despite learning this maneuver, you may still not feel as though foods taste as they did before your surgery. Over time, however, generally within the first 6-9 months, most laryngectomees feel as if their foods taste "normal" again.

Stoma Care

Once healed, the tracheostoma should not require any particular care. In the event mucous crusting occurs, these crusts should first be softened with water or saline and wiped away. Many patients find the use of long handled tweezers helpful in removing mucous crusting but care should be taken to not pinch or damage the tracheal mucosa. If you are experiencing frequent crusting, your SLP can assist you with management.

Cleaning any noted debris from the stoma in the morning is typically all that many patients will require although routine removal of mucous during the day is normal.

Using Suction

The use of suction is common during the immediate post-operative period. During this time, forceful coughing may be difficult and there may be a degree of general deconditioning that occurs in the days immediately following your surgery. For this reason, suction is often helpful.

It is, however, very important to begin to learn to cough and clear your secretions without the use of suction. Many patients often believe they will require the use of suction the rest of their life, although this is not true. In fact, in most cases, we discourage the use of suction once there has been adequate post-operative recuperation. Your doctor and SLP will reinforce this concept, and help to wean you from the use of suction, if necessary.

A forceful, effective cough serves to help clear secretions that are lower in the air passages of the lungs. When a person uses suction to clear secretions, there is typically not the same force applied during coughing. The deeper secretions are not as effectively cleared, may accumulate, and ultimately prove to be *more* difficult to clear. It is very important you begin to learn to clear your secretions without the help of suction. There are cases, however, where prolonged suction use may be necessary and those cases are managed individually.

Bathing and Water Activities

After your laryngectomy, it is very important that you protect your stoma from water getting into it. The open stoma serves as a direct "pipeline" into the lungs. During showers, you can wear a special cover that is designed to keep water away from the stoma. Your SLP can provide information about how to obtain this device. Taking a bath is not generally recommended; however, should you choose to sit in a tub of water, be sure to keep the water level no higher than your navel.

Recreational activities such as swimming, boating, fishing and other water sports are not advised after your surgery as they represent a significant drowning risk. There are, however, centers that specialize in adaptive equipment to allow laryngectomees to participate more safely in these activities. The speech pathology department can assist you with this information should you choose. Without proper adaptive equipment, however, it is strongly advised you avoid such activities following your laryngectomy. With a laryngectomee stoma, should you fall into water, your lungs can fill with water within seconds. You should also always be very cautious when walking near deep water, such as on docks.

Swallowing After Laryngectomy

Many patients have reported it is harder to swallow following their laryngectomy surgery. That may be true. How the swallow works after a laryngectomy is very different from how someone with a larynx will swallow.

With the larynx in place, there are several structures in the throat that assist in the swallow process. Many of these are removed during the laryngectomy surgery which means how you swallow really is different. And in some cases, this can take some time to adjust.

During the laryngectomy surgery, many of the structures in the throat, useful in swallowing before the surgery, are removed. This does not mean a laryngectomee cannot swallow but the process of swallowing is certainly different.

This is very important to remember. **A laryngectomee will not choke** or strangle, even if it feels as if the food is "stuck" in the throat. Anxiety over a fear of choking may create more tension in the throat and make it even more difficult for the food material to pass.

Many patients and family members are often questioning how a laryngectomee can swallow once all the "parts" have been removed. Its important to understand that swallowing is very different following a laryngectomy, but it can also be very effective.

Practice and proper instruction can often speed the process of returning to a more normal diet and way of eating.

Radiation, as well as flap reconstruction, can both negatively impact the strength and effectiveness of the throat muscles. In many cases, therapy can help improve the overall strength and effectiveness of the swallow, although this will first need to be evaluated by the speech pathologist.

The cricopharyngeus is also impacted as a result of the laryngectomy surgery. The structures used to pull this muscle open, allowing food to pass into the esophagus, have been removed. Many times, a *myotomy* is performed during the laryngectomy surgery, which serves to relax the uppermost region of the esophagus, including the cricopharyngeus and thus, eases the passage of food through this region.

Smelling after Laryngectomy

Following a laryngectomy, the sense of smell, or *olfaction*, remains intact. In a standard laryngectomy surgery, there is no impact from the surgery to the nerves of olfaction that allow for smelling scents, aromas and odors. What *has* changed, however, is the pathway of airflow during respiration. Prior to the laryngectomy, air would flow into the body through the nose and mouth. This movement of air through the nose allowed for scents and aromas to be detected as the smells came in contact with the tiny nerve endings in the nose that are responsible for the sense of smell.

Following a laryngectomy, however, there is no longer an active flow of air through the nose during breathing. This can be perceived as a loss of smell.

The "polite yawn technique" has become a standard in helping laryngectomees regain their capacity to smell. With this technique, you create a vacuum within the upper airway. This serves to draw air into the nasal passages and by doing this, the sense of smell is then enhanced with the new airflow.

It is known as the "polite yawn" technique because the movements involved are similar to those when you attempt to yawn with a closed mouth. Swift, downward movement of the lower jaw and tongue, while *keeping the lips closed,* will create a subtle vacuum, drawing air into the nasal passages.

With practice, you will be able to achieve the same vacuum using more subtle (but effective) tongue movements. Your SLP can be very helpful in providing training of this technique.

Tracheoesophageal Voice Prosthesis (TEP)

A tracheoesophageal voice prosthesis is a device made of medical grade silicone, which is positioned within the "party wall" which is the shared wall between the trachea and the esophagus. The voice prosthesis itself does not produce a voice. The purpose of the prosthesis is to allow air to be delivered from the lungs into the esophagus where it is expelled through the mouth. The passage of air as it travels from the esophagus to the mouth, results in vibration of tissues in the lower pharynx, or throat, producing sound which serves as the new voice for laryngectomy patients.

These devices function through the use of a one-way valves The valve serves to open as air flows through, then should close completely when speech is over to ensure food and liquid from the esophagus are not allowed to enter the trachea.

Although many advances have been made over the years, these devices, once placed, are not permanent and will require periodic replacement. How long a voice prosthesis lasts depends on many factors and varies greatly from patient to patient. Your SLP is highly skilled in helping you to achieve the longest lifetime of your voice prosthesis and may modify your routine care and/or diet to assist with achieving longer device life as needed.

Cleaning Your Voice Prosthesis

Most patients now use an indwelling-type voice prosthesis. This type of prosthesis is placed either in the operating room or in the office by your SLP and designed to be self-retaining (meaning, it is meant to stay in position until it is purposely removed). These are the latest in the evolution of low-maintenance voice prostheses.

It is very important, however, that these prostheses be properly cleaned to ensure proper function as well as the longest lifetime of the valve.

At the time of the initial prosthesis placement, you will be provided with a brush and a flush. The prosthesis should be cleaned twice a day, morning and evening, although intermittent cleaning during the day is also appropriate to assist with the function of the voice prosthesis as needed.

The brush serves to loosen debris and biofilm from the prosthesis. Once loosened, the flush rinses this material away. Using both the brush and the flush will assist in prolonging the life of the voice prosthesis and ensuring it is functioning properly.

Using an Adhesive Housing

An adhesive housing is the most common way laryngectomees use peristomal devices. These adhesive 'baseplates" are designed with a universal 22mm hub opening which serves as a means of securing most laryngectomy stomal supplies and accessories such as HMEs, tubes and shower guards. There are several varieties of adhesive housing, all designed to meet the unique and different needs of each patient. Your SLP will determine which version is most appropriate for you, and this may change as the surface of your neck changes with continued healing and/or aging.

Using an HME Cassette

The acronym HME is short for: "Heat & Moisture Exchange." These small cassettes are positioned over the stoma and designed to have all the air you breath pass through them, -both inhaled air and exhaled air.

Although your throat has been drastically changed through the laryngectomy surgery, your lungs have also had quite a transition from being disconnected from your upper respiratory tract. Being a neck breather changes the dynamics and physiology of how you breathe. Through the use of an HME, the lungs are receiving air more similar to when you were breathing through your nose. This is especially important in preventing mucous crusting and plugging as well as to ensure your secretions are well managed.

We are designed to breathe humidified air. Prior to the laryngectomy, the air you were breathing was moistened by passing through the humid passages of the nose and throat. The laryngectomy surgery, however, disconnects the upper airway passages from your lungs and all the air you breath now enters your lungs through the neck. As a result, this air no longer has the benefit of first receiving humidification or warmth before entering the lungs. This drier air serves to thicken secretions, contribute to crusting in the airways and can also stop the lungs' natural ability to move secretions out.

By using an HME, you are helping to restore much of what the nasal passages used to do for humidifying and heating the air you inhaled. When in place, the HME cassette will trap the moist and warm air you exhale (think of fogging a mirror with your breath). The foam inside the cassette is treated with a special salt that is designed to retain moisture in the humid air you exhale, as it passes through the HME. It will also capture the warmth of the air you exhale. Then, as you inhale, the air passes back through this warm and moist foam, which helps it to be similar to the air you were inhaling through your nose before the laryngectomy.

HMEs are very helpful in secretion management as well as prevention of mucous plugging. Wearing and HME 24/7 will ensure optimal respiratory physiology following a laryngectomy.

There are different versions of HMEs and your SLP will determine which is best appropriate for you. It is very important HMEs are used and worn properly. Improper use may mean you do not get the maximum benefit toward your pulmonary rehabilitation. Similarly, there can be risks to your health.

Proper Use of an HME Cassette:

- It should be worn everyday, all day 24/7.
  - Exceptions are during mucous removal from the cassette or during showering.
- The HME cassette MUST BE REPLACED **EVERY 24 HOURS**
- If you feel you are unable to breath well through the cassette, promptly remove and clean.

Cleaning Mucous From An HME

It is very normal to cough and clear secretions throughout the day. With continued use of an HME, these secretions should become more manageable, Many patients notice the amount of secretions diminishes and they become less thick. This will not happen overnight and several weeks may be required to notice this change.

When mucous is coughed, it will rest against the back of the HME cassette were plastic bars known as "mucous guards" are preventing the mucous from deeply penetrating the foam. When this happens, it may become difficult to breath until the mucous is removed. It is important, therefore, the clear the mucous from the HME cassette as often as necessary to ensure you are breathing comfortable and your secretions are well managed.

Proper Cleaning of the HME:

- Remove the cassette, holding the housing firmly in place so as not to dislodge in any way.
- Using a tissue or soft cloth, simply wipe the mucous off the cassette.
- A soft toothbrush can be used to help clear thicker mucous if necessary.
- NEVER RUN YOU HME CASSETTE UNDER WATER, NEVER IMMERSE IN WATER (this may wash out the antimicrobial component that is essential to its function)

Larytube Use and Cleaning

A Larytube is a pliable silicone tube, designed to maintain an airway of a laryngectomy. It has a curvature consistent with the curvature of the trachea following a laryngectomy. Larytubes are designed to be used with an HME cassette and can be used with either an adhesive housing, or ties/clips. Larytubes can also be worn with a TEP, allowing you to speak normally. Your SLP will determine the appropriate tube for you to use, if/when necessary.

A larytube is used to ensure there is adequate support of the stoma as it heals following surgery. Primarily, it helps to keep the airway open in the presence of any post-operative swelling that may exist. During your first SLP visit as an outpatient, your SLP will assess the overall condition of your stoma and will help to wean you from the tube. In most cases, a tube is not necessary following post-operative recovery. There are special circumstances, however, when a tube may be indicated even after you are fully recovered from surgery. It is VERY IMPORTANT that you use the tube as directed by your SLP if it is determined you should wear one.

TEPs and HME's During Radiation Treatment

Voice Prostheses During Radiation

Although many patients are worried about the effects of radiation to their voice prosthesis. Radiation will not harm the voice prosthesis in any way. Despite this, many patients find it too painful to speak during the later stages of radiation. Although the voice prosthesis may not be used for speaking, it is important to continue cleaning it as you normally would.

HME Use During Radiation

Regular use of an HME is very important to achieve the maximum benefit from the device. This is especially true during radiation when there can be some changes to the tracheal lining causing it to bleed easily with any crusting. There can also be changes to the thickness of the mucous you are producing and the HME will help to ensure your secretions are more manageable. For this reason, you should continue to wear your HME at all times, most especially during radiation.

Although it is important to continue wearing your HME, wearing an adhesive housing is not recommended during radiation. Since it is important to continue wearing the HME cassette, your SLP will assist you in finding the best alternate method for housing your HME cassette. Usually, you will be provided with a Larytube for this purpose. Like the other devices, the Larytube is not impacted by the radiation. It can also serve to provide support to the stoma during treatment and recovery, when the tissues can become very irritated and swollen.

Laryngectomy FAQs

Why am I coughing so much mucous?

Coughing as a neck breather means anything you should expel air from your lungs through your stoma. Although you are accustomed to covering your mouth when you cough, you will learn instead to cover your stoma. Initially following surgery and for several weeks thereafter, you will cough a great deal of mucous and secretions from your lungs. The lungs are increasing the output of secretions and mucous in response to the changes in you anatomy and physiology. Regular application of the HME assist with restoring normal lung function by delivering the filtered and humidified air the lungs are accustomed to. Over time with regular HME application, the secretion production will slow down.

Many patients are concerned to see, despite regular HME application and sufficient healing from surgery, they continue to cough mucous from their stoma. It should be stressed that that lungs normally produce mucous in healthy, non-laryngectomized people as a protective layer to help keep lung tissue moist as well as to serve to trap inhaled particles that may be harmful to lung tissue. In a non-laryngectomized patient, these secretions are coughed frequently during the course of a normal day and typically swallowed. Following a laryngectomy, however, these secretions must be expelled from the stoma and wiped away. Having to more directly manage these secretions can easily lead one to believe there is "more than normal" production, when in fact, this is a healthy lung function. It is important to remember this is quite normal, although your doctor or SLP may be able to offer suggestions for improved secretion management if it seems atypical.

When can I get a TEP?

In many cases, the TE puncture is created at the time of the laryngectomy surgery. In some cases, the prosthesis is placed at the time of surgery but other times, the prosthesis is placed in the office as an outpatient after a period of healing (typically no more than 2 weeks). In the event you do not receive a TE puncture during your surgery (usually due to more extensive surgery/reconstruction), you will be punctured after a period of sufficient healing, usually around 3-4 months after surgery.

How often/when do I use and HME?

In order to be of maximum benefit, the HME should be worn 24 hours per day, every day of the week. During periods of increased physician activity, should you notice a sense of restricted breathing, remove the device until respiration becomes more comfortable. This should only be done for more emergent cases. For regular increased physical activity, the speech pathology staff can help select the most appropriate HME for use which would (hopefully) allow for continued utilization, even during these periods of increased respiratory demands.

How often do I replace my HME cassette?

The HME cassette needs to be replaced every 24 hours. It is never ok to use these beyond the 24 hour device lifetime, nor is it appropriate to attempt to wash the HME. These should also never be run under water or immersed in water as this may wash away the antimicrobial agent that is essential for adequate HME function

Although the HME cassette is treated with an agent to help prevent bacterial growth, after 24 hours the cassette needs to be replaced to ensure it does not begin to develop bacterial colonies.

When do I use my Larytube?

The Larytube is designed to stabilize the stoma, particularly during the post-operative recovery and healing phase following surgery. Using the Larytube ensure the airway is maintained, even in the presence of healing tissues and potential post-op inflammation and swelling. Typically speaking, this should be worm 24/7 until indicated otherwise by your doctor or SLP. Often times, the speech staff will "wean" you off the Larytube, seeing how well you do without it. Most patient, following sufficient post-operative recovery time, do not need to use the Larytube.

There are cases, however, where a patient has a stoma that shrinks spontaneously when left without a tube. In those cases, the Larytube may be used regularly, despite adequate and normal post-operative recovery. Your SLP will determine if the Larytube is necessary for regular use or note.

I can't wear my adhesive housing during radiation so how do I continue wearing my HME cassette?

During radiation the skin on the neck can become very sensitive and applying/removing the adhesive housing may become very uncomfortable. Your SLP can provide you with a Larytube or Larybutton to use during radiation. This will serve to hold the HME cassette as well as provide stomal support during radiation.

Is it ok to wear my adhesive/HME during hyperbaric oxygen treatments?

There is no contraindication for wearing the adhesive housing or HME during hyperbaric oxygen treatments, although facility regulations may require you to remove it during your treatment.

Can I keep my voice prosthesis if I am going to have hyperbaric oxygen treatments?

Yes. The voice prosthesis can remain in place throughout the duration of your hyperbaric oxygen treatments.

Why do I need to change my HME cassette every 24 hours?

Although the HME cassette is treated with an agent to help prevent bacterial growth, after 24 hours the cassette needs to be replaced to ensure it does not begin to develop bacterial colonies.

How often do I change my adhesive housing?

Unlike the HME cassette which must be changed every 24 hours, an HME housing can be worn as long as the adhesive seal is functional. If using a TEP, this means changing the adhesive housing when excessive air leaks are noted. If not using a TEP, the housing should be changed when there is no longer a sufficient seal against the skin.

Why can't I smell?

Following a laryngectomy, the sense of smell, or *olfaction*, remains intact. In a standard laryngectomy surgery, there is no impact from the surgery to the nerves of olfaction that allow for smelling scents, aromas and odors. What *has* changed, however, is the pathway of airflow during respiration. Prior to the laryngectomy, air would flow into the body through the nose and mouth. This movement of air through the nose allowed for scents and aromas to be detected as the smells came in contact with the tiny nerve endings in the nose that are responsible for the sense of smell.

The "polite yawn technique" has become a standard in helping laryngectomees regain their ability to smell. See "Smelling After a Laryngectomy."

Why can't I taste my food like I used to?

Because our sense of taste is strongly related to our sense of smell, you will notice that foods may no longer taste the way they did before the surgery. The tongue is able to detect five basic tastes: sweet, sour, salt, bitter and savory. Our sense of smell adds to the taste of our food and allows us to recognize the difference between steak and pizza, for example. Once you start eating after surgery, you will notice that your favorite foods may taste quite different from what you remember.

The technique the speech pathology staff will teach you is also referred to is the "polite yawn technique." Its works to help move air through your nose, and by doing this, will also improve your ability to taste more accurately. Many laryngectomees have reported this helps foods taste more "normal." Despite learning this maneuver, you may still not feel as though foods taste as they did before your surgery. Over time, however, generally within the first 6-9 months, most laryngectomees feel as if their foods taste "normal" again.

Why is it harder to swallow?

During the laryngectomy surgery, many of the structures in the throat, useful in swallowing before the surgery, are removed. This does not mean a laryngectomee cannot swallow but the process of swallowing is certainly different.

This is very important to remember. **A laryngectomee will not choke** or strangle, even if it feels as if the food is "stuck" in the throat. Anxiety over a fear of choking may create more tension in the throat and make it even more difficult for the food material to pass.

Many patients and family members are often questioning how a laryngectomee can swallow once all the "parts" have been removed. Its important to understand that swallowing is very different following a laryngectomy, but it can also be very effective.

Practice and proper instruction can often speed the process of returning to a more normal diet and way of eating. Radiation, as well as flap reconstruction, can both negatively impact the strength and effectiveness of the pharyngeal constriction. In many cases, therapy can help improve the overall strength and effectiveness of the swallow, although this will first need to be evaluated by the speech pathologist.

References:

1.	Edge SB, Byrd DR, Compton CC, Fritz AG, Greene FL. *AJCC Cancer Staging Manual*. 2010.

2.	Colevas AD. Population-based evaluation of incidence trends in oropharyngeal cancer focusing on socioeconomic status, sex, and race/ethnicity. *Head Neck*. 2014;36(1):34–42. doi:10.1002/hed.23253.

3.	Pfister DG, Spencer S, Brizel DM, et al. Head and neck cancers, Version 2.2014. Clinical practice guidelines in oncology. *J Natl Compr Canc Netw*. 2014;12(10):1454–1487.

4.	Piccirillo JF. *Cancer Patient-Specific Prognostic Information*. 2001.

5.	Schmidt RL, Hall BJ, Layfield LJ. A systematic review and meta-analysis of the diagnostic accuracy of ultrasound-guided core needle biopsy for salivary gland lesions. *Am J Clin Pathol*. 2011;136(4):516–526. doi:10.1309/AJCP5LTQ4RVOQAIT.

6.	Agulnik M, McGann CF, Mittal BB, Gordon SC. Management of salivary gland malignancies: current and developing therapies. *Oncology ....* 2008.

7.	Fleming ID, Cooper JS, Hensen DE, Hutter RV. *American Joint Commission on Cancer (AJCC) Staging Manual*. 1997.

8.	Haugen BR, Alexander EK, Bible KC, Doherty G. 2015 American Thyroid Association Management Guidelines for Adult Patients with Thyroid Nodules and Differentiated Thyroid Cancer. *....* 2015.

9.	Gaissert HA, Mark EJ. Tracheobronchial gland tumors. *Cancer Control*. 2006;13(4):286–294.

10.	Urdaneta AI, Yu JB, Wilson LD. Population based cancer registry analysis of primary tracheal carcinoma. *Am J Clin Oncol*. 2011;34(1):32–37. doi:10.1097/COC.0b013e3181cae8ab.

11.	Velez Jo ET, Morehead RS. Hemoptysis and dyspnea in a 67-year-old man with a normal chest radiograph. *Chest*. 1999;116(3):803–807.

12.	Grillo HC, Mathisen DJ. Primary tracheal tumors: treatment and results. *The Annals of thoracic surgery*. 1990.

13.	Suzuki T. What is the best management strategy for adenoid cystic carcinoma of the trachea? *Ann Thorac Cardiovasc Surg*. 2011;17(6):535–538.